ADHD 2.0

FOR ADULTS

Essential Coping Strategies to Control Impulsiveness,

Improve Social & Work Commitments Organization,

and Break Through Barriers.

Margaret Hampton

Table of Contents

Adhd 2.0 & Social Anxiety For Adults

Adhd 2.0 Effect On Marriage

About the Author

Margaret Hampton is an author, cognitive behavioral counselor, and speaker with more than 20 years of clinical practice. Her books have impacted the lives of adults with ADHD every day. They offer a comprehensive look into ADHD, including everything from real-life stories to management tools and advice for dealing with a close person who has ADHD.

Besides being professionally involved in the topic, Ms. Hampton is also an ADHD individual herself and her children. She has extensive work and knowledge in recognizing and coping with ADHD.

At her conferences, Ms. Hampton always offers timeless, research-backed advice and solutions applicable to adults and children. She highlights the most significant challenges and combines traditional treatment with contemporary treatment.

Mrs. Hampton, within her books, proves that ADHD can be an invaluable asset in one person's life and she proves it throughout many examples. She has become an amazing painter herself, as a consequence of her neurodiversity's imagination and creativity, turning a disorder into a little life achievement.

ADHD 2.0
&
SOCIAL ANXIETY
for Adults

The 7-day Revolution

Overcome Attention Deficit Disorder.

Social Skills | Self-Discipline | Focus Mastery | Habits.

Win Friends & Achieve Goals to Success.

Introduction

If you put me at a big celebration, business, or charity event, I will instinctively walk toward the people in the room who have ADHD. This is not on purpose. It simply occurs that way. It isn't because I have the expertise and wrote this book or because I've worked in this sector for more than 20 years. It's not because two of my three kids have ADHD. It's because I intuitively recognize my community. I, too, suffer from ADHD, but you probably wouldn't see it initially.

Unless you know where to look, the signs of ADHD are generally invisible. Most people wouldn't realize that I have trouble sitting because I don't fidget much and don't get up and walk about when I do not need to. Instead, I keep myself entertained by wearing jewelry that I can fiddle with or follow the ridges of the glass with my palm. In social circumstances, you might not see all of the ways I'm trying to fit in or that it takes a lot of work to appear "normal."

I am always working hard to hide my ADHD inclinations by seeming to care about polite small conversation, not interrupting others, and intently listening. I have been thinking about my behavior for years. It is wrong! I had to make something, a change that would help me overcome my issues and be better, not make me hide my inclinations. So yes, this book is also about social anxiety or the anxiety that comes from ADHD.

The combination of appearing to be an adult and hog-tying random thoughts and acts eventually leads to social tiredness. So I gravitate toward those who are mischievous and interruptive like myself. Discussions with other people who have ADHD swing around various themes in a freestyle flow of consciousness. I'm no longer trying to blend in. I'm not very concerned with ADHD symptoms. I'm in the moment, loving the party, getting to know my ADHD self, and relieving the anxiety I feel.

You might not realize how ADHD impacts me daily unless you spend time with me. You may notice that I struggle to recall things, pay attention in meetings, listen to instructions, and complete activities. You're highly likely to observe me searching for missing objects while muttering, "Now, where might that be?" If you don't know that there are indications of ADHD, you could dismiss me as careless, disorganized, untrustworthy, or even stupid. People frequently misinterpret ADHD symptoms as character qualities rather than neurological anomalies.

I know a lot of people do not understand ADHD. I also know that they misunderstand the signs they perceive. I try to appear "normal," which necessitates me faking it. Every day, I struggle with seemingly straightforward activities in life. For example, I'd want to call and meet a friend for coffee, but anything that isn't already occurring seems too big to organize. Some days, I feel I can't gather my scattered ideas long enough to begin a task, remain on track, and complete it.

My attempts to suppress my symptoms frequently fail horribly. Little ADHD mistakes accumulate during the day: I double-book customers, struggle to pay a bill, or leave my vehicle windows open on a wet day. I'm fatigued and feel like a failure by the evening, and I'm sure others perceive me as a failure.

I'm all too aware of how those of us with ADHD are seen by the non-ADHD world. Previous bosses, acquaintances, and even family members have misinterpreted my symptoms as carelessness, sloth, or incompetence. Even when others are aware that I have ADHD, they frequently link my symptoms to character defects, asking me to pay more attention to this or that.

I routinely talk to various organisations about the effects of ADHD on individuals. I spoke to a large group of parents about parenting emotionally stable ADHD children on one such occasion. I stressed the significance of teaching their children problem-solving skills during the lesson. I described how quickly people with ADHD experience feelings of guilt and inadequacy. Following that, some of the parents formed a queue to ask further questions, and I assisted the participants in developing their next steps in parenting. At the stage, a well-meaning non-ADHD parent approached me and said, "I'll have your glass. I'm sure you'll forget to do it," then grinned and laughed. I must have appeared surprised since she came to a halt and asked, "Did you need this glass?" Her comments had hit me square in the face. She'd thought I'd forget and made a joke out of my difficulties, delivering the all-too-familiar jab, "I'll do this for you since you're too careless to do it." I had previously planned for my carelessness by placing the remote control I was using next to the glass so I wouldn't lose it.

I thought about how quickly I might feel incompetent on the way home. I hoped the woman had just stated, "I would be delighted to take care of this for you." I know she didn't try to deliver the negative impression that I was irresponsible, but people with ADHD are bombarded with these subtle signals. They accumulate and create dents in our feeling of well-being.

Part of the difficulty stems from how people see me, but another aspect is how harshly I criticise myself. I am sensitive to criticism and judgment, as are many people with ADHD. I make the cognitive error of seeing criticism where it is not intended, like with the helpful parent at the meeting.

I've attempted to conceal my natural way of thinking or behaving from others to fit into a non-ADHD environment. To assist me in blending in, I researched the characteristics of non-ADHD people's thinking and behavior. I've decided that I can no longer pretend to be neurotypical. Instead, I need to be open about how ADHD impacts me, how I think, and how I behave, and then utilize that knowledge to assist me in navigating the environment in which I live. It's a never-ending game of adapting, but it works! I don't have to act any longer. I recognize that I am unique compared to people who do not have ADHD. And – despite living in a fast-paced, complex world full of interruptions – I can navigate by constantly gaining new skills and attitudes. Learning how my brain works allow me to devise hacks and workarounds to get things done and be kind to myself when I don't.

If you have ADHD, you must understand that your brain is not damaged. Your brain is wired differently and does not function similarly to a "normal" or neurotypical brain. Compared to the non-ADHD brain, some portions of the ADHD brain are hyperactive, while others are underactive. Understanding, accepting, and compensating for our differences is much easier when we see how the ADHD brain differs from the neurotypical brain.

The realisation that ADHD is a complex condition that impacts all aspects of a person's life is the first step in managing it. I hope you will learn to recognize your ADHD habits and make the required adjustments to live productively. The information you will receive will help you live more efficiently. The knowledge you will receive about ADHD will allow you to manage your symptoms without having to fake them to others or yourself.

Why should I expect this book to be helpful to me?

This question is valid; however, as with many topics with ADHD, the answer is complex.

To begin, the majority of the coping strategies I will address in this book are likely to be similar, if not the same, to those found in the numerous popular publications that advise on managing adult ADHD.

ADHD is not a lack of information problem; instead, it is a productivity problem—being unable to execute what you set out to do consistently.

Second, since ADHD is a problem with skill performance, the resemblance of coping methods and practices across various books and programs and the repeated information is not bad. To be more specific, having numerous and varied remembrances of these techniques helps to refresh the significance of these routines in your life constantly.

The combination of skill review and somewhat diverse presentations of these concepts across multiple mediums adds a level of freshness and offers new perspectives on old themes. The diversified presentation of ideas and teachings, just as in learning, enhances the possibility that these notions will "stick" and come back up during everyday life when you need them the most. Diet and fitness books routinely rank among the top sales each year – not because earlier books did not give valuable advice – because changing these behaviors is tough.

In terms of your willingness to adapt, my method expects a lot from you. Coping methods and take-away notes are important tools, but they are not unchanging laws of physics. You must employ them so they can be effective. You must be willing to confront and suspend your concerns about your power to transform and reduce your social anxiety.

Chapter One: Understanding ADHD

This chapter focuses on ADHD and all the general information you need to know. This information will assist you in determining whether or not the step-by-step methods and techniques featured in this book are appropriate for you. You will learn how to comprehend the features of adult ADHD, discover why ADHD symptoms persist in adults and understand that ADHD is a genuine adult diagnosis.

Attention deficit/hyperactivity disorder (ADHD) is a recognized medical and mental condition. ADHD manifests itself in childhood, and many children with ADHD have significant symptoms as adults. People experience three basic types of signs: poor focus, hyperactivity, and impulsivity.

Many individuals with ADHD have at least some hyperactivity, poor attention, and impulsivity, while many people have symptoms predominantly from one group. Attention Deficit Disorder (ADD) is used when an individual has selective attention symptoms but not hyperactive symptoms.

People with ADHD can develop coping techniques to help them deal with the problems that come with the disorder. ADHD is a neurological illness that has nothing to do with intelligence, aptitude, laziness, being insane or not, and so on. The treatment plan – which usually begins after an individual takes ADHD drugs for many months – can help adults regulate their ADHD symptoms. You will see big changes if you actively study skills and practice them regularly.

A mental health practitioner will usually diagnose ADHD based on the definition of the American Psychiatric Association's Diagnostic and Statistical Manual of Mental Disorders (DSM). The DSM, besides anxiety disorders, features bipolar disorders, feeding and eating disorders, depressive disorders, and compulsive personality disorders. The DSM-5 includes all of the different mental illnesses and the symptoms and other criteria that an individual must exhibit to be diagnosed with them.

Individuals must demonstrate at least five of the nine potential inattention symptoms and/or five of the nine potential impulsivity/ hyperactivity symptoms to fulfill the DSM- 5 criteria for adult ADHD. Individuals with ADHD – mostly inattentive presentation – show five or more symptoms in the inattention group.

ADHD – mainly impulsive/ hyperactive presentation – is defined as five or more symptoms in the impulsivity/hyperactivity group (Hallowell, 2022). Those who have five or more symptoms from both groups have ADHD with a mixed presentation. The inability to pay attention to details, trouble sustaining attention in tasks, appearing not to listen when spoken to immediately, failing to adhere to commands, problems with organization, denial of activities that require prolonged mental effort, regularly losing things, easily confused, and forgetfulness are all examples of inattentive symptoms. Fidgeting, departing one's seat repeatedly, feelings of restlessness, inability to participate in peaceful tasks, being "on the move," chatting incessantly, blurting out replies, having difficulties waiting in lines, and constantly interrupting are all hyperactive/impulsive symptoms.

Furthermore, the person must have had at least some of the symptoms before 12, and the symptoms must be present in approximately two different situations. The symptoms must interact with the person's ability to act, and another mental disorder must not better explain the symptoms.

15

How Do We Tell the Difference Between ADHD and Normal Functioning?

Some of the symptoms described above sound normal. Most individuals would undoubtedly admit to being easily distracted or having difficulty organising themselves. This is true for a large number of mental illnesses. For example, everyone experiences sadness from time to time, but not everyone fits the criteria for clinical depression.

To be diagnosed with ADHD, an individual must be experiencing severe difficulty in some element of their life, such as job, school, or interaction patterns. In DSM-5, there is a greater emphasis on impairment particular to adults, such as impairment at work.

In addition, ADHD must drive the person's suffering and disability and not by another illness to qualify for the diagnosis. A comprehensive evaluation is required to eliminate the possibility that the symptoms result from another psychological disease.

How Do Cognitive and Behavioral Factors Contribute to Adult ADHD?

Cognitive components (thoughts and beliefs) might exacerbate ADHD symptoms. For instance, if a person is confronted with something he would find overwhelming, he may divert his focus elsewhere or say things like, "I can't do this," "I don't want this," or "I will do this later." The behavioral components are what people do that might aggravate ADHD symptoms. Actual behaviors might include delaying doing what you should be doing or maintaining or discontinuing an organizing structure.

It is no secret that the primary symptoms of ADHD are biological. Nevertheless, researchers think cognitive and behavioral factors also influence symptom levels (Hallowell, 2022).

Core neuropsychiatric deficits limit successful coping beginning in childhood. Adults with ADHD have been suffering from the illness since infancy. Distractibility, disorganization, trouble following through on activities, and impulsivity are all characteristics that can impede individuals with ADHD from learning or practicing appropriate coping techniques.

Individuals with this disease generally have chronic underachievement or other experiences that they may characterize as "failures." Due to this history of failure, individuals with ADHD may acquire unduly negative ideas about themselves and negative, dysfunctional thinking while approaching activities. The negative thoughts and attitudes might contribute to avoidance or attention deficits. When presented with tasks or issues that they find difficult or dull, individuals with ADHD divert their attention even more, and accompanying behavioral symptoms might worsen.

Does Medication Treat ADHD Successfully?

Yes. Medications are presently the first-line therapy option for adult ADHD, and they have received the greatest research attention. These drugs fall into four categories: stimulants, monoamine oxidase inhibitors, tricyclic antidepressants, and atypical antidepressants.

However, a significant proportion of people who take antidepressants (about 20% to 50%) are nonresponders. A nonresponder is someone whose symptoms are not adequately lessened or who cannot tolerate the drugs. Furthermore, those considered responders often demonstrate a decrease in just 50% or fewer of the primary symptoms of ADHD (Hallowell, 2022).

Thanks to these findings, guidelines for the optimal treatment of adult ADHD include combining psychotherapy (particularly cognitive-behavioral therapy) with medicines. Many of the main symptoms of ADHD, such as focus issues, hyperactivity, and impulsivity, can be reduced with medication.

Adult ADHD Is A Real Medical Condition

ADHD in adulthood is a real, reliable medical disorder that affects up to 5% of people in the United States. Adult ADHD has always been a contentious diagnosis. One explanation for this is that psychiatric diagnoses are difficult to validate. Specialists can do blood work, x-rays, biopsies, or even take a patient's temperature to aid in making a diagnosis in many different medical professions. In some circumstances, overt medical proof supplements the patient's narrative.

However, for psychological problems, these tests are currently impossible. Doctors must diagnose psychiatric diseases solely on their patients' self-reported symptoms, their observations of the patient, or the views of others. Psychiatrists and psychologists have devised a method for classifying mental diseases by examining groupings of exhibited symptoms.

Sufficient scientific data has been collected over the last few decades, concluding that ADHD is a genuine, substantial, stressful, interfering, and valid medical disease. This data includes proof that ADHD can be diagnosed reliably in adults (Hallowell, 2022) and that the diagnosis fulfills diagnostic validity requirements comparable to those of other psychiatric illnesses. Key symptoms in adulthood include difficulties with attention, inhibition, and self-regulation. These basic symptoms result in adult limitations such as the following:

- Poor school and work performance (difficulty with the organization or making plans, becoming distracted, insufficient sustained attention to reading and documentation, procrastination, poor time management, and rash decision making).

- Impaired interpersonal skills (e.g., friendship problems, poor follow-through on responsibilities, poor listening skills, various difficulties with intimate relationships).
- Problems with behavior (for example, those with ADHD end up less educated, have issues with money management, have difficulty managing their house, and have chaotic routines).
- Medication treatment research and genetic investigations that include adoption and family studies, neurochemistry research, and neuroimaging provide additional support for the validity of ADHD as a diagnosis.

ADHD affects between 1% and 5% of individuals. This percentage is comparable with estimations that ADHD affects (Weiss & Hechtman, 1993) 2% to 9% of school-age children, and follow-up studies of ADHD children suggest that debilitating ADHD symptoms remain into adulthood (beyond puberty) in 30% to 80% of diagnosed children.

The ADHD People

A problem child that makes its parents insane by being completely disorganized, incapable of following through on almost anything, not capable of cleaning up a room, doing household chores, or performing just about any given task; the one who is constantly interrupting, looking for excuses for a job not done, and usually operating far below potential. We're the child who gets lectured regularly about how we're squandering our skills, squandering the great chance that our intrinsic aptitude offers us to succeed, and failing to use what our parents have given us properly.

We are also the talented executives who consistently fall short due to missed deadlines, forgotten duties, social faux pas, and squandered chances. We are too frequently the addicts, misfits, jobless, and criminals who are just one diagnosis and treatment plan away from turning our lives around. We are the individuals for whom Marlon Brando declared in the famous 1954 film On the Waterfront, "I could become a contender." So many could have and should have, been contenders.

But we can also make amends. We are the seemingly uninterested meeting attendee who appears out of nowhere with a novel idea that saves the day. We are frequently the "underachieving" adults whose ability blossoms with the proper type of assistance and achieves impressive success despite a shaky school record. We are the competitors as well as the winners.

We're also creative and dynamic instructors, preachers, circus performers, stand-up comedians, Navy SEALs or Army Rangers, innovators, tinkerers, and trend setters. There are self-made multimillionaires among us, Pulitzer and Nobel prize winners, Academy, Grammy, Tony, Emmy award winners, top-tier trial attorneys, neurosurgeons, commodities market traders, and stockbrokers (Weiss & Hechtman, 1993). And we are frequently business owners. We are businessmen, and most adult ADHD patients we meet are or desire to be business owners. Dan Sullivan – the founder and owner of a business assistance organization called Strategic Coach – has ADHD and believes that at least half of his customers have ADHD.

Because individuals with ADHD don't stand out from the crowd, our disease is almost unnoticed. However, if you were to crawl into our thoughts, you would find a different scene. Ideas would fly around like kernels in a popcorn machine, rat-a-tat rapidly and on no discernible schedule. Ideas come in random, unpredictable spurts.

20

Since we can't turn off this specific popcorn machine, we're frequently unable to halt the formation of ideas at night. Our thoughts never seem to rest.

Indeed, our brains are here, there, and just about everywhere simultaneously, which occasionally emerges as the appearance of being someplace else, in some dreaming condition. It is not a secret that we frequently miss the metaphorical boat, but maybe we should construct an aircraft or get a pogo stick instead. We tune out during a job interview and don't get the job, but perhaps we spot a poster in the human resource department waiting area that inspires a fresh idea that leads to a patented innovation.

We upset others by forgetting names and commitments, but we make amends by recognizing something no one else has noticed. We shoot ourselves in the foot only to invent a painless means of removing the bullet on the spot. "It can be the individuals' no one can envision anything of who perform the things no one can imagine," stated the famous mathematician Alan Turing. That describes us.

ADHD is a more prosperous, more intricate, precarious, and possibly beneficial state of being than neurotypical people would believe and what diagnostic tests (Weiss & Hechtman, 1993) would have you believe.

The word "ADHD" refers to a manner of being in the world. It is a collection of characteristics unique to a particular type of mind and may be a significant benefit based on how a person controls it.

After covering ADHD, and its essential features, we need to focus on something else. As someone with ADHD, you probably already know "anxiety." I also think that you know the word social and how it is related to anxiety. Let's learn what social anxiety is and what the two of them can do to someone.

Chapter Two: Social Anxiety

Social anxiety is a catch-all phrase for the dread, uncertainty, and worry that most individuals experience from time to time in their interactions with others.

Individuals with social anxiety claim to be shy and may have been shy their whole lives, while some individuals who are not shy also struggle with social anxiety. Individuals face social anxiety when they believe they will do something mortifying or disappointing.

Social anxiety makes you think that other individuals are evaluating you negatively because of anything you said or did. The dread of doing anything embarrassing or humiliating is restricting. It also makes one feel self-conscious and aware of the likelihood that one may do something embarrassing or humiliating.

Who would want to engage in conversation if they knew it would only disclose their awkwardness, inadequacies, or inclination to blush? Socially anxious people often believe that their encounters with others will be excruciatingly revealing. Others will see their flaws or discomfort and reject, ignore, criticize, or dismiss them for not acting more acceptably (Stein, 2008).

When you see things this way, it's tough to communicate naturally with others, and it's difficult to chat, listen, or form friends. It frequently leads to isolation and loneliness. For many individuals, one of the most heartbreaking aspects of having this disease is that it stops them from being intimate with others or finding a partner with whom to spend their lives.

Socially anxious individuals are frequently friendly to others and have a fair share of the good attributes that others value. They may have a sense of humor, be active and kind, generous and understanding, serious, humorous, quiet, or vivacious, and they act in various ways naturally when they are at ease.

However, because feeling at ease in company is difficult for the socially anxious and causes them anxiety, these attributes are frequently hidden from view. Their fear hampers their capacity to communicate themselves, and their ability (Stein, 2008) to do so may have been rusty due to lack of use. Indeed, socially apprehensive individuals may have lost faith in their appealing traits and self-confidence.

One of the benefits of learning to manage social anxiety is that it helps you express previously inhibited elements of yourself, allowing you to appreciate – rather than dread – being yourself. Finally, it teaches you to trust yourself rather than mistrust yourself since you realize that no one's social behavior is faultless and everyone makes errors. Mistakes are acceptable; they are a natural part of being human, and there is no need to let them derail you.

Identifying the issue

Definitions are essential because they help us focus on the aspects of social anxiety caused by ADHD that create discomfort and prolong the anguish.

Anxiety about social situations is common. Everyone experiences it at some point (so everyone understands it). It would be insane for us to believe that we would never experience social anxiety again. Seeking a complete cure would be trying the impossible. Instead, it is beneficial to begin by defining when social anxiety becomes an issue if you have ADHD and then understand the factors that contribute to it persisting.

As you'll see in the next chapters, concentrating your efforts on improving these things – particularly learning how to be less self-conscious – may make a tremendous impact. It alleviates pain and suffering and allows you to live the life you want. But first, you must comprehend the concept of social anxiety.

The American Psychiatric Association's Diagnostic and Statistical Manual (Stein, 2008) defines the type and level of social anxiety that qualifies someone for a diagnosis of social anxiety related to ADHD. The guidebook outlines four major criteria:

1. Persistent apprehension about one or more social or performance circumstances in which the individual is exposed to new individuals or may be scrutinized by others. The individual is afraid that they would act unpleasant and humiliatingly (or exhibit anxiety symptoms). It is important to note that individuals with social phobia may not do something humiliating or unpleasant; they only fear that they will. Their symptoms don't even have to be visible. They merely need to consider the prospect of something happening to become afraid and nervous.
2. Exposure to dreaded social settings nearly always causes anxiety, like talking on the phone, approaching a crowded room, or speaking publicly in front of others. While there is not a hard and fast distinction between normal and clinical anxiety levels, there are various levels of social anxiety.
3. The individual knows that their dread is unwarranted or excessive. One of the most problematic aspects of having social anxiety disorder due to ADHD is knowing that what makes you worry is not harmful and may not affect other people. But understanding that you suffer "irrationally" and

"excessively" in comparison to others and that your pain is in some ways unwarranted simply makes it worse. It might leave you feeling insecure, nervous, incompetent, or inferior.

4. Fearful circumstances are avoided or endured with great worry or pain. It's only natural to avoid or flee from terrifying circumstances. The sensation of terror warns you of the probability of danger, and staying might be dangerous. On the other hand, people who suffer from social anxiety are tough since they do not want to be isolated and lonely. They have no control over the origins of their fear. Interaction with others – such as shopping, traveling, or working – cannot be avoided entirely. Socially anxious individuals, like everyone else, want to work, make friends, and feel like they belong. Rather than avoiding or fleeing tough situations, people may tolerate these stressful situations despite their misery, focusing on keeping the dangers or hazards as low as possible and keeping themselves as secure as possible. Because of the severity of their worry, this technique appears only logical.

Whether or not these features of the condition are severe enough to meet diagnostic criteria is, to some part, a question of professional judgment, as there is no hard and fast rule for determining what level of suffering counts as substantial. Dreading public speaking is the most prevalent fear mentioned by individuals with social anxiety disorder caused by ADHD (75% of people with this diagnosis are terrified to speak in public). However, one of the most commonly listed anxieties is the fear of public speaking. It is, in fact, more frequent than the fear of death.

Social anxiety can be divided into two types (Stein, 2008). For some, social anxiety is restricted to a few settings, such as dining in public or being among sexually attractive individuals; for others, it is more likely to influence most scenarios requiring interaction.

Because there is no clear and fast line between being socially anxious and having a medically diagnosable disease, this book will use the everyday usage of social anxiety rather than 'social anxiety due to ADHD.'

The Connection Between ADHD and Social Anxiety

It's important to realize that ADHD affects many individuals — around 4.4 percent (Rodebaugh, Heimberg & Holaway, 2004) of American adults and up to 10% of American adults children. The same is true for social anxiety, which affects an average of 12.1% of Americans at some point in their lives.

Social anxiety is a mental health diagnosis characterized by worry or anxiety about social circumstances in which others may scrutinize the individual. Typically, the individual is terrified of acting in a humiliating or unpleasant manner, which would result in rejection. Individuals with social anxiety virtually always experience discomfort in social interactions, and they frequently avoid social events entirely due to worry or pain.

According to the CDC, children with ADHD are more likely to have additional mental health issues such as anxiety, stress, depression, and autism spectrum disorder, making social connections more challenging.

The CDC also reports that approximately one in every ten children with ADHD has anxiety. According to a 2015 study, there is a relationship between social anxiety and ADHD. Anxiety and ADHD are typical co-occurring disorders, and social anxiety and ADHD are not rare.

When people are uneasy or anxious in social situations, they may want to touch items or fidget with their fingers. This uneasiness in social situations is also frequent among people with ADHD. Once they are required to concentrate or sit still, they may fidget.

ADHD never travels alone, and social anxiety is a familiar companion. Social anxiety may severely hinder professional and academic performance and relationships, whether you can't consume food around others, avoid cafés or stores due to stranger discussions, or despise public speaking.

Many ADHD teenagers and young adults have social anxiety due to executive functioning issues with emotional regulation, learning and memory, and self-awareness. People who suffer from social anxiety may avoid specific triggering scenarios such as in-person classes, while others may feel extremely uneasy and awkward in any social setting (Rodebaugh, Heimberg & Holaway, 2004).

An intense dread causes social anxiety that others criticize you so harshly that their replies will crush you. When you are preoccupied with the negative judgments of others, you are unable to be yourself, form great connections, or construct a fulfilling life. Instead, social anxiety stymies you at every turn.

ADHD | SOCIAL ANXIETY

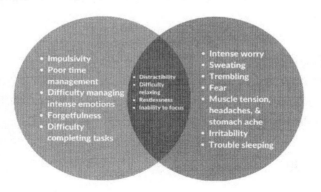

(Cuncic, 2021)

The Signs and Symptoms of Social Anxiety

The Venn Diagram describes the four major categories of ADHD and social anxiety. No two individuals are the same, and there are several possible symptoms, so if the ones you are experiencing are not present, simply add them to the list (Rodebaugh, Heimberg & Holaway, 2004).

To begin assessing the problem for yourself, consider how your interpretation of social anxiety impacts your thoughts, behaviors, body, and emotions. It would be odd not to have any symptoms in any of these four different categories, but some of them might be difficult to recognize at first. Spend some time thinking about your specific experience with social anxiety, using this list as a suggestion.

Examples of social anxiety indications and symptoms

1. **Effects on thoughts**
- Concerning yourself with what others think of you.
- Difficulty concentrating or remembering what others say.
- Concentrating your focus on yourself and being very aware of what you do and say.
- Considering what may go wrong ahead of time.
- Ruminating about an event after it already happened to examine if you did anything wrong.

2. **Effects on behavior**
- Speaking fast or silently, muttering, or mispronouncing words.
- Avoid seeing someone by taking precautions to ensure that you do not draw attention to yourself.
- Keeping safe by avoiding awkward social circumstances or scenarios.

3. Physical effects

- Anxiety symptoms visible to others, such as flushing, sweating, or shaking.
- Tension: the aches and pains that come from not being able to relax.
- Panic attacks: hammering heart, dizziness or nausea, or shortness of breath.

4. Effects on emotions

- Anxiety, fear, apprehension, and self-consciousness.
- Frustration and rage directed towards oneself or others.
- Feelings of inadequacy and lack of confidence.
- Feeling down, dejected, or despairing about your ability to change.

In practice, the symptoms interact in diverse ways, such that ideas, behaviors, physiological reactions, and emotions (or feelings) all impact one another. For example, believing you look silly makes you feel self-conscious, so you turn aside and attempt to blend into the background, which causes you to become aware that you are shivering and your heart is pounding. Or, since you're sweaty and panicked, it's challenging to think of what to say, so you blurt out something that makes no sense, and then you feel ashamed.

How Does It Feel To Have This Problem?

A description and a list of symptoms are good places to start when thinking about social anxiety, but they don't give the whole picture or explain the pain involved. It is not unexpected that a disease that can touch many facets of life should have far-reaching consequences.

Subtle kinds of avoidance:

While some socially anxious individuals avoid going out with friends, attending meetings, or attending social occasions like weddings, others continue to attend events they fear. This participation gives the impression that they are not fearful of these situations, but this ignores the numerous subtle ways one might avoid disagreeable circumstances, such as speaking gently or hurrying on. It is critical not to ignore subtle forms of avoidance since they play a significant role in perpetuating the issue like other forms of avoidance. Below are a few more examples.

Subtle kinds of avoidance examples

- Waiting for somebody else to arrive before entering a crowded room.
- Putting things off, such as visiting the neighbours or shopping during peak hours.
- Turning aside when you notice someone is approaching who makes you nervous.
- Refusing to discuss anything personal.
- Not using your hands if you believe that people are looking.
- Refusing to eat in public places.

Behaviors that promote safety

Other people are a source of anxiety for those who are socially anxious, and one of the issues with other people is that you never know what they will do next. They may, unwittingly, touch you at any time, make you feel weird by asking you a specific question, introduce you to someone who makes you feel most anxious, ask for your viewpoint, or simply walk away from you to speak to someone else. When you're with other people, you can feel constantly threatened, and it's not easy to figure out what you should do to stop feeling bad. In these scenarios, your mind instinctively shifts to thinking about how to be safe.

Socially anxious people create safety behaviors or things they do to decrease their sense of being at risk, such as looking at the floor to avoid eye contact, wearing make-up to conceal their blushes, or leaving the room as soon as a meeting is over, so they don't have to engage in small talk. Below are some more instances of safe practices.

As you read through the list below, you will see that some of them appear to be opposed – such as being silent or attempting to continue the discussion – but this is because different people desire to do various things to feel safe.

Some people feel comfortable saying little and making sure that what they say makes sense. These behaviors give them the impression that they are less likely to make a fool of themselves. Some feel safer if they take charge of keeping a discussion going. It might feel safer to keep talking when quiet feels like an eternity, even if you're not making any sense.

Safety behavior* examples

- Rehearse what you're about to say and mentally double-check that you've got the words correct.
- Speaking slowly or softly or speaking quickly and not pausing to take a breath.
- Putting your hands to your mouth or hiding your hands or face.
- Tightening your grip or locking your knees together to control shaking.
- Allowing your hair to fall in front of your face, wearing loose-fitting clothing, attempting to amuse others by telling jokes, or never risking telling a joke.
- Not talking about yourself or your thoughts; refraining from expressing your ideas.
- Saying nothing that may be construed as challenging or contentious; always agreeing with others.
- Wearing clothing that will allow you to blend in.
- Keeping close to a safe person or in a safe location; not taking any chances.

- Looking for the exit route whenever you are out in public.

Safety behavior is anything you do to keep yourself safe. Many safety behaviors entail avoiding unwanted attention.

Dwelling on the issue

Social anxiety may strike at any time and can feel overpowering, partially because of the uncertainty of others and partly because the dread of it is continually in mind. Anticipating worry contributes to the problem. When I think about future meetings, I think about how things may go wrong, typically in mysterious and terrifying ways.

Even after an incident, the mind remains vulnerable to increased worry by repeatedly replaying ideas, pictures, and recollections of what occurred. Socially anxious people tend to fixate on parts of their relationships with others that bother them. People who suffer from social anxiety perform post-mortems based on what they believe happened rather than what actually occurred, on what they believe other people thought of them rather than what they actually thought.

Self-esteem, self-confidence, and inferiority feelings

Social anxiety provokes different negative reactions and actions. Often you feel as if you are less promising than others or more strange, which affects your self-esteem and self-confidence.

You start to expect people to reject or ignore you, and you interpret their actions – such as the way they look at you or talk to you – as signals that they dislike you. You are afraid of becoming the target of their criticism or unfavorable appraisal or of being found wanting in some manner as if someone will expose your flaws or deficiencies.

As a result, you may have a persistent undertone of terror, as if you are lurching from one lucky escape to the next. Some socially anxious individuals believe that if others knew what they were truly like, they would abandon them altogether. Social anxious individuals will go to extraordinary measures to disguise their "true selves" even if nothing is problematic with them other than feeling nervous.

Of course, this makes it difficult for them to convey an opinion or communicate how they feel about something. They may also believe that other individuals are never socially anxious, that they have less – or less socially revealing – flaws and shortcomings, or that they can go through life without worrying about what others think of them. In reality, being impervious to others produces just as many issues as being too sensitive to them.

Frustration and anger; demoralization and sadness

It feels difficult to suppress elements of your character, so it's no surprise that social anxiety may depress you after a time. When it conflicts with doing the things you want to do and being the kind of person you want to be, knowing you can be around people brings a slew of other emotions. You may feel demoralized, sad, nervous, bitter, and frustrated that others seem to find so many things simple that you find difficult. Anxiety is not the sole emotion linked to social anxiety.

Performance consequences

The problem with excessive anxiety levels is that they disrupt activities and the capacity to carry out plans. They make it more difficult for individuals to perform to the best of their ability and impede them from accomplishing their goals. A certain amount of worry is beneficial if you have to go to an interview or take an exam as it may energize and encourage you and help you concentrate your attention. Too much anxiety, however, becomes a distraction and makes it difficult to act normally or do your best. This anxiety might also make it difficult for people to know you. Social anxiety prevents individuals from doing what they desire and are capable of accomplishing. This may have a wide variety of diverse implications on professions, personal relationships, friendships, jobs, and leisure activities in the long term.

The following illustrates how social anxiety can affect someone:

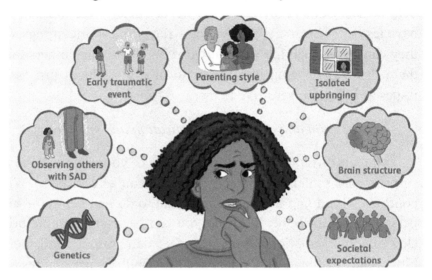

(Cuncic, 2021)

Social anxiety may be restricted to one significant life element– such as eating or speaking in public – but it is more often associated with broader and more widespread impacts. Some individuals do well at work until they are promoted to a position that requires them to be more "visible" or supervise others. They may be unable to accept the promotion because it requires them to attend meetings where they must account for their department's operations or give presentations, attend a training program, or organize, monitor, and assume responsibility for the work of others. These individuals may decline advancement and stay in professions well below their talents, so they fail to realize a large portion of their potential.

Others may function effectively at work – even in high-profile professional occupations or socially demanding – such as sales or

34

public relations. These individuals have few issues as long as workplace customs shelter them. They are okay in the lab, computer room, or operation theatre, but they may feel lost in unplanned social events or when their position is not clearly defined. They find it difficult to establish acquaintances and have a hard time making small talk (Koyuncu, Ertekin, Yüksel, Aslantaş, Ertekin, Çelebi, Binbay & Tükel, 2015). Despite their professional success, they may still feel isolated and lonely, and their social anxiety may cause them to miss out on chances to build deep and personal connections.

Many people suffer from what is known as dating anxiety. This anxiety is common enough to be considered entirely normal, and people go through these agonies when they find someone good-looking. They cannot do the things that will help them get to know the person they feel strongly about.

Others have one or two close friends and feel most at ease in the company of individuals they know well, like when they are with their spouses or encircled by their family. Social anxiety makes it difficult for them to meet new people, move to new areas, or find new methods to please themselves, and their lives may become severely confined and constricted.

Chapter Three: ADHD and Social Anxiety - The Endless Connection

Anxiety is a common disorder in the general population, but it is more prevalent in those with ADHD. Their comorbidity rates are estimated to be approximately 25%. Nonetheless, these figures imply that most people with ADHD do not have accompanying anxiety issues, but this is not our clinical opinion.

Studies often use strict cut-offs that put a person in or out of a certain group. These studies are useful in identifying people who have a comorbid anxiety disorder with a degree of functional impairment. Nevertheless, many people may not legally satisfy a type of disease. Still, they arrive with anxiety issues, which generally arise (Koyuncu, Ertekin, Yüksel, Aslantaş, Ertekin, Çelebi, Binbay & Tükel, 2015) from previous experience and a lack of confidence, which may impede their progress in therapy.

ADHD and anxiety comorbidity rates are associated with the similarities between ADHD and anxiety symptoms (restlessness, lack of attention, unceasing mental activity). Furthermore, a 25% overlap has been documented in community and clinic research, indicating that comorbidity rates are unlikely to merely reflect symptoms being 'counted' twice in around one-quarter of cases.

Anxiety is described as a side effect of stimulant medications in certain circumstances. When this occurs after treatment, it may be beneficial to urge a mental assessment and potential switch to non-stimulant medication.

Perinatal issues – such as late pregnancy difficulties, problems after birth, and the neonatal period – have been identified as risk factors for comorbid ADHD and anxiety, especially in individuals without a family history of ADHD. Consequently, many people enter the world predisposed to develop nervous and maladaptive coping techniques.

These maladaptive coping techniques manifest because of repeated criticism from others (both actual and imagined), which causes people to be frightened about completing activities or entering settings. Adults with ADHD may develop "anticipatory anxiety" about circumstances in which they have previously encountered disappointment and/or failure due to disadvantages in academic success, failure in the job, and difficulties getting along with others.

People with anxiety and ADHD may become fixated with their previous behaviors and/or performance and worry about future occurrences and interpersonal performance. Individuals may relive unpleasant memories, such as when they think they have done poorly, when they believe others have assessed them to be 'below standard' compared to others, and moments of shame due to mistakes of judgment and/or improper behavior.

Anxiety is likely to manifest itself in various ways in ADHD adults. People with ADHD are more prone to be self-conscious or vulnerable to shame or humiliation.

Most individuals with ADHD experience anxiety in school as 'performance anxiety,' such as when they have to get up in class and read aloud. They make typos, misspell words, and sometimes skip whole sentences. Their classmates ridicule or bully them or mock and call them names. In such circumstances, people may retreat or rashly strike out. In any case, this has a detrimental social impact, and ADHD young adults lose their capacity to engage comfortably with their classmates (Koyuncu, Ertekin, Yüksel, Aslantaş, Ertekin, Çelebi, Binbay & Tükel, 2015).

Some young adults overcompensate by striving to satisfy everyone or bullying other kids. Others make up for it by being the class clown. They may seek friendships at school from children outside of their peer group or prefer adult company.

Small fears grow into larger anxieties over time, compounded as individuals go from school into early adulthood and face higher scholastic and social obligations. The early nervous ADHD kid has evolved a method of interacting with the environment built on uncertainty and uneasiness before they even know where they are. Anxiety becomes widespread, undermining their views and confidence in their ability to succeed in almost whatever they undertake. This anxiety sometimes leads to a preoccupation or over-concern about their ability to perform numerous jobs and areas of function.

In today's culture, a person's work, home, or car they drive symbolizes their success. There are several expectations to meet, necessitating the capacity to multitask and take on different duties and positions. Whether your title is mother, father, wife, spouse, daughter, son, friend, church member, youth leader, advisor, manager, worker, or executive, you must juggle these positions and your other responsibilities. It might seem like there are many plates spinning in the air. Society is fast and hectic, and individuals with ADHD prefer speed above precision, so when they work quickly, they make mistakes and fail.

Everything else one needs to think about or accomplish becomes considerably more difficult when one is worried. Anxiety influences cognitive processes by influencing the assessment and evaluation of events, resulting in an internal shift of emphasis to excessive self-monitoring and self-regulation.

Anxiety worsens attention problems and impulsivity. It may impair one's capacity to reason. As a result, ADHD people – who already have cognitive weaknesses – will become even more susceptible to anxious circumstances by functioning less effectively. For someone with generalised anxiety disorder, this means they get a "double dosage" of cognitive impairments since ADHD symptoms become much more prominent when they need to concentrate the most. This anxiety makes ADHD evaluation more difficult since these individuals get agitated at the testing site.

Many cognitive tests begin with straightforward tasks and grow progressively more difficult to measure individual variations in strengths and limitations. This increase in difficulty implies that a person will inevitably reach a point when they cannot answer a question or solve a puzzle.

This testing technique may confirm existing notions that they are "stupid" or may have them relive terrible school memories. Individuals who get very worried are less likely to perform effectively and are more likely to abandon assignments, leading them to fall short of their potential and the tester to underestimate their level of performance. Children with comorbid anxiety and ADHD perform worse on activities requiring short-term or working memory, i.e., tasks requiring both active processing and transitory information storage.

Anxiety may redirect resources away from storage and processing within the working memory system. However, it is theorized that anxiety serves a motivating purpose by increasing arousal, which may enhance attentional control. This increased arousal is more likely to happen in activities that do not need knowledge retention (i.e., memory processing) but require the person to block a response, such as continuous performance or stop tasks.

Children with ADHD and accompanying anxiety may do better in such activities. Unfortunately, there has not been any research on people with comorbid ADHD and anxiety.

Anxiety disorders may manifest themselves in various ways, including generalised anxiety, social phobia, simple phobia, phobias, panic disorder, obsessive-compulsive disorder, and post-traumatic stress disorder. Individuals with ADHD are more likely to have generalised anxiety, but individuals (Koyuncu, Ertekin, Yüksel, Aslantaş, Ertekin, Çelebi, Binbay & Tükel, 2015) have also reported social phobia, panic disorder, and obsessive-compulsive disorder.

These are not mutually exclusive categories, and ADHD adults may have difficulties. Difficulties may be more visible depending on the social, academic, or vocational obligations, as well as their life history at the moment (Koyuncu, Ertekin, Yüksel, Aslantaş, Ertekin, Çelebi, Binbay & Tükel, 2015). For example, depending on the scenario, a person may have generalised anxiety difficulties and social phobia, and in times of extreme stress, they may also suffer panic symptoms.

People with ADHD may develop social anxiety subsequently to their overall concern about everything and everyone they meet. Feeling different from their peers causes some people to compare themselves to others on a frequent and unfavourable basis, resulting in them selectively responding to their own perceived bad attributes and the good characteristics of others.

Some individuals may regularly need reassurance in social settings, such as "Did I come across okay?" or "Was I not diplomatic?" They feel self-conscious and awkward because they are concerned that others are watching them in social situations. Some individuals attempt to compensate by behaving foolishly and becoming the "heart and soul of the party." In such cases, anxiety treatments should aim to reduce anxious thoughts, feelings, and behavior and calm the individual so that they do not respond in an overly excited manner. This calming allows the person to avoid drawing undue attention to themselves by behaving in a bizarre and/or inappropriate manner (which others may perceive as childish). This is not to reduce individuals with ADHD's innate inventiveness and passion but to urge the individual to act with greater control and maturity.

Because the incidence of ADHD is greater among people with Tourette's syndrome and the rate of Tourette's is higher among those with ADHD, the increased prevalence of the obsessive-compulsive disorder in those with ADHD may be mediated by its linkages with Tourette's syndrome. Obsessive Compulsive Disorder (OCD) symptoms are also likely to exacerbate attention problems by shifting available resources to obsessive thoughts.

Symptoms connected with OCD, on the other hand, may be tactics adopted by individuals with ADHD to compensate for an attention deficit by checking for mistakes or items they may have forgotten. However, when a person's anxiety level rises, this checking behavior may become more repetitive and compulsive (Koyuncu, Ertekin, Yüksel, Aslantaş, Ertekin, Çelebi, Binbay & Tükel, 2015). Individuals may be embarrassed by their private obsessions or compulsions, which may prompt them to avoid discussing them with doctors, especially during their evaluation. They may believe that by treating their ADHD, their OCD symptoms will go away.

Over-focusing in an obsessive or perseverative manner may lead to task failure owing to excessive concentration on a small part of a job. Some people who struggle with these issues may choose not to undertake a job rather than risk doing it badly. Exploration and questioning concepts and rigorous desensitization are effective therapy techniques for reducing repetitive checking behaviors.

Because ADHD symptoms and anxiety symptoms overlap, it is critical to conduct a thorough and comprehensive evaluation of the anxiety-related problem and determine the relationship between the individual's thoughts, beliefs, feelings, and behaviors regarding their ability to complete a task or perform competently in a situation. As with standard cognitive behavioral anxiety therapy, a psychoeducational component explaining the anxiety model and the link between cognition and behavior is essential.

Assessment

Before we jump onto possible solutions, let's look at this questionnaire:

Check how often you have experienced the following symptoms:	Never	Occasionally	Sometimes	Often	More than often	Always
General Anxiety						
I have worried about money, paying bills, and debts.						
I have worried about not being able to finish work/ tasks/ school assignments.						
I am worried about my health.						
I am worried about the future and things going wrong.						
I am worried that I have failed as a parent/ employee/ son/ daughter.						
Social Anxiety						
I am self-conscious.						
I avoid social events.						
I avoid crowds.						

I am worried about performance.							
I am worried about meeting other people.							
Panic							
I have felt a constriction in my chest.							
I have felt heart palpitations.							
I thought I was having a heart attack.							
I felt dizzy, and I fainted.							
I feel the blood rushing around my head.							
Obsessive-compulsive disorder							
I felt uncomfortable if the house was not tidy or clean.							
I need to check everything several times.							
I have to do things in a routine; otherwise, I become worried.							
I tend to over-focus.							
I had intrusive thoughts.							

The anxiety checklist is introduced above and crafted around concepts frequently discussed as a cause of anxiety by individuals at clinics (generalized anxiety, social anxiety, panic, obsessive-compulsive issues) to assist the client and therapist in identifying the subtype of the comorbid presenting problem of anxiety.

Thus, the anxiety checklist (Koyuncu, Ertekin, Yüksel, Aslantaş, Ertekin, Çelebi, Binbay & Tükel, 2015) serves as a helpful guide for determining whether anxiety problems are general or specific. It also serves as a foundation for conversation and exploration, allowing you to take an adaptive treatment approach and fundamentally plan and structure treatment. However, anxiety classifications are not mutually exclusive.

Treatment

When treating people with ADHD and chronic anxiety vs. treating individuals without ADHD who have anxiety, there are two major differences:

1. Recognize the overlap in anxiety and ADHD symptoms and try to separate the best treatment symptoms by the approaches recommended in the following chapters to improve attention and decrease impulsivity.
2. Because ADHD people have trouble deferring pleasure, it is critical to implement an instant reward system to positively reinforce success and performance on a much more regular basis than is now used.

The suggested treatment models are based on critical steps of the therapy process: cognitive behavioral psychoeducation on the anxiety model, learning to deal with negative thoughts, developing self-control, and modifying behavior.

Chapter Four: What Do You Have to Do?

We discussed the current concept of Attention-Deficit/Hyperactivity Disorder (ADHD) as an issue connected to executive function or motivational deficiencies in Chapter 1. Executive functions constitute the self-regulation that enables you to select and complete activities across time to attain personally meaningful goals.

The problem for most individuals with ADHD is not a lack of objectives or desire, but rather that ADHD interferes with the constant follow-through on the stage process procedure over time to attain those goals, particularly when the result does not (Çelebi & Ünal, 2021) come quickly enough. For instance, we all want to be in better physical condition, but it may be tough to stick to a daily regimen of eating healthier and exercising until we get the desired effects.

Adults with ADHD find it even more challenging to break down long-term or significant objectives into step-by-step strategies and then continuously implement these plans. To that aim, it is essential to establish precise and explicit plans throughout the day.

These intentions aid in the organisation and movement of your day. This is especially true on days (such as the weekend) or periods of the day when you lack the structure offered by your job, school, or other regular responsibilities. You may be self-employed, a graduate student focusing on a thesis, or a stay-at-home parent, all of which require you to create your own schedule to a considerable extent. The fourth chapter will go through how to use a daily planner to organize and arrange your schedule. For the time being, your responsibility is to define the exact activities you will complete on a given day that, when combined, will build the structure for your day.

Task selection and prioritising, and providing a framework for your day represent how you choose to "spend yourself," including your commitment of time, energy, and effort. There will be a plethora of tasks to sift through, including somewhat basic domestic duties (taking out the trash), vital errands and tasks (grocery shopping, paying bills), leisure, cultivating connections, and other important personal pursuits (exercise, work, school).

This chapter aims to explore the to-do list as a tool for identifying, sorting through, and prioritising the numerous necessary chores and activities in your life. To make the to-do list manageable and functional, we will distinguish between complete and daily to-do lists and talk about how to prioritize and increase the chances of completing chores. The first stage in the process is to make a plan and schedule time to do so.

Time for Planning

Although we are just getting started with the concept of "having time to plan," it will be a recurring problem for managing time and other coping skills throughout this book. Planning is a commitment that needs an initial commitment of time and effort—often much less than you expect—for higher profits later in the day, week, and month—often much more than you wish.

Living with ADHD and anxiety involves time and effort, which is inevitable. Most individuals with ADHD and anxiety believe that others do not have to go through all these processes to manage their day. This viewpoint may provoke a long-held feeling of being different from others or act as a justification for not devoting time and effort to working on a to-do list which can be perceived as "unnatural"

46

or "strange." Because of this feeling, you resist making an effort to start a to-do list and tell yourself that you'll be able to handle all your daily tasks without a to-do list. Sadly, frequently failing to plan results in the feeling that you do not achieve anything meaningful at the end of the day.

In reality, most non-ADHD and anxiety individuals organize (Çelebi & Ünal, 2021) their days and utilize some version of a to-do list. Someone who does not have ADHD and anxiety may be able to avoid writing down or going back to their work lists, and their follow-through looks to be easy. These people have most likely established habits that need less effort to maintain, but everyone spends some time and effort organising their day.

This book suggests devoting an "honest" 10 minutes to working on the planning activities outlined below in terms of what to accomplish. Working on the to-do list requires just an electronic word processing file or worksheet, a smartphone's notepad function, or simply (and arguably the best approach) paper and pen.

The more clear and definite your strategy for planning, the better. We recommend that you designate a particular location where you will sit to work on your to-do list at a realistic time of the day or when you will have at least 10 minutes to dedicate to it. Adults with ADHD and anxiety may express being distracted by other ideas or having difficulties concentrating at first, so we recommend a 600-second time commitment—the "honest" 10 minutes – until planning becomes a habit. This time range allows you to participate in and finish the activity and "remember to remember" what you need to accomplish.

The previous phases are designed to put you in a position to create your strategy. You should strive to use the same location each day at the same time to spend your 10 minutes planning (Hallowell,

2022). The concept may be modified to the situation, especially if you cannot use the same location to plan your to-do list.

To prioritize and create a list of things to do on a given day, you must first comprehend the many duties, responsibilities, and commitments that supply you with a laundry list of possibilities. The next section covers the function of the complete to-do list.

You must:

1. Devote 600 seconds or 10 minutes to planning.
2. Find an area free of distractions.
3. Plan your day for 10 minutes (600 seconds).
4. Make a note of your intentions in your daily planner.
5. Define to-do items using strong, behavioral phrases for what you want to "do."

A Complete To-Do List

The complete to-do list is what its name implies: a complete list of your many activities, obligations, and projects. It is also known as a "dump list" of everything required. The attempt to remember multiple responsibilities throughout the day, with several extra ones "popping into mind" at inconvenient times (Hallowell, 2022), such as the awful, too-late recollection of things forgotten ("Oh no, my friend's birthday was yesterday and I forgot it!"), as well as those foreboding issues that randomly pop up but are not yet urgent ("Valentine's Day falls on a Friday; I should make dinner arrangements sooner rather than later.").

Instead of attempting to remember everything, the complete to-do list is an externalized and customized record of everything you need to do. The list serves two purposes: first, to provide a method for thinking through and unloading these duties, and second, to provide a lasting record of them so that you do not have to recall and keep the list in your thoughts constantly.

Based on your specific situation, you will decide how "complete" you want your list to be. For the most part, your complete list will span the next one to six weeks, with things about the next week taking precedence on your daily list. However, there may be approaching events that demand immediate attention, such as holiday plans, business travels, or school or work assignments that cannot be put off until the last minute.

It is also helpful to think through some activities that do not have a timeframe but are characterised as tasks to be completed shortly or other activities that are currently low priority but will become important in the future.

"It is too daunting for me to think about and confront all I have to accomplish every day" is a frequent response to the concept of the complete to-do list. We understand that it is daunting, so you should get it out of your mind, write it down, and store it for future reference. The complete to-do list allows you to write down and organize these random activities and thoughts, so you do not forget to complete an essential task.

The complete to-do list should be reviewed regularly to help you recall and identify priorities and integrate new activities and commitments that may have emerged since the last review. You are not expected to create a new to-do list every day; rather, this is an exercise to help you focus on your most critical short-, mid-, and long-term chores over the next six weeks or so. However, many people find it beneficial to sit down at times to review and update their lists or spend some time starting a new to-do list to get a grip on what needs to be done in the coming several weeks.

You must:

1. Get a notebook or open a word document to keep track of your complete to-do list.
2. Find an area free of distractions.
3. Make a list of your duties, plans, chores, commitments, leisure ideas, and so on for the next one to six weeks (or whatever period works best for you). This list is your "dump list."
4. Keep your notebook or word document close to you.
5. The complete to-do list reminds you of activities and responsibilities without depending on your memory. Refer to it regularly for useful reminders of things you can accomplish, but this is not your daily to-do list.

Daily To-Do List

The daily to-do list – as the name suggests – is a daily list that provides a personalised collection of activity reminders that are important to you. You don't need a reminder to get to work, but you will need to make a particular business-related phone call or dedicate time to a report throughout your workday.

To-do activities are duties that demand a concentrated effort from you to complete throughout the length of a regular day, such as shopping, booking a medical appointment, meditating, or doing a specific household activity (such as unloading the dishwasher). You can use this list to specify particular responsibilities in various jobs.

The point of the list is to record all your outstanding duties, while the daily to-do list is intended to be an easy-to-access, disposable list of activities for today. We recommend writing the list on a little index card that may be kept in your pocket or other easily accessible position (like posted on a computer display or other conspicuous location).

The modest size of the note card should keep the work list reasonable, with our advice being to start with two or three activities (and certainly no more than five) to prevent feeling overwhelmed. Phones and other electrical gadgets include notepad functions that are simple and helpful. An old-fashioned paper version is still a faster and simpler method to retrieve and refresh your memory (Hallowell, 2022). Writing down the list by hand boosts task encoding and prepares you for behavioral follow-through. In any case, you must choose a simple format to use and manage.

Another general rule for creating the daily to-do list is to specify tasks in precise, behavioral terms to maximise the chance of completion. For instance, you may have a list item that reads "clean up the kitchen." Even though this is a personally meaningful chore, when phrased as such, it becomes too daunting since it includes multiple smaller tasks (empty dishwasher, load dishwasher, wash down counters, clean inside of the microwave, arrange cabinets, and so on). You may not know where to begin, which increases tension, and finally allows you to postpone the chore, generally with a comfortable but ultimately self-defeating justification like "I'll check my email, and then I'll be in the mood to fix the kitchen."

The ability to split enormous tasks into components is an important coping skill mentioned in subsequent chapters. This talent is not a surprise to anybody with ADHD and anxiety, but this list allows you to put it into practice in precise ways. As previously shown, "clean up the kitchen" may be more clearly and behaviorally defined as "load dishwasher and place clean dishes where they go," or whatever starting action seems achievable to you at the time ("I will empty the bowls").

It's okay if you finish that work and opt not to do anything else. You may add another kitchen-related job to your daily to-do list for the following day. On the other hand, most individuals with ADHD and anxiety have observed that once they get started, they generally stay moving" and will add additional tasks to their list.

The first precise and behaviorally defined activity is meant to stimulate and engage you by making the first step reasonable, similar to wading into the shallow end of a swimming pool. This first step gets you started, and you'll probably wind up doing more than you expected since the work isn't as awful as you thought it would be.

Construct a Strategy

Making a daily to-do list and checking it throughout the day can help you stay on top of these priorities. Each review and reminder exposes you to something you would normally avoid and prepares you for action rather than allowing these vital chores to fall victim to poor recall or engagement in diversions.

The reminder to enter the room with a strategy is a good motto to keep your priorities front and center while performing your tasks. One of the difficulties of ADHD and anxiety are resisting the want to do something more exciting but less significant than what you set out to achieve.

Entering a room with a strategy requires reminding oneself of the purpose of entering the room, storing or accessing a computer file, or doing any other activity included in your immediate task plan. When you obtain something for a project or transition between chores, you are open to distraction.

Entering the room with a strategy provides you with a goal to strive toward, such as not clicking on the Internet icon while opening a computer file for a work assignment ("I am going to work on the report until 2 pm, and then I can start playing games.")

This coping mechanism may also assist you in returning to a task when you find yourself wandering at home or work when you want to be productive ("I came downstairs to grab paper for the printer. I'll collect it and return upstairs to continue my job").

It is critical to anticipate typical triggers for distraction and flight from work and devise proactive strategies to cope with them.

You   *must:*

Daily To-Do List

1. Locate a piece of paper, the back of an invoice, or another piece of throwaway paper.
2. Devote ten minutes to creating your daily to-do list.
3. Your daily to-do list consists of tasks that are not on your regular schedule but demand a particular commitment of time and effort.
4. Keep your list to a maximum of two to five things. When in doubt, go on the side of fewer things rather than more—you can always add more after you finish them.
5. Specify tasks in behavioral terms or acts you can "do."
6. Determine a reasonable time period for completing each activity.
7. Use your daily planner to identify periods throughout the day when you will "appoint" yourself to do each assignment.
8. Complete each assignment on time and cross it off the list.

Enter the Room with a Strategy

1. Explain why you're entering a room (or workplace, sitting at a desk, etc.). What is your objective, and why is it important to you?
2. Specify the behavioral steps or activities you will do in the room to begin the activity and behave per your aims.
3. How do you become "off track"? What may jeopardise your plans? Predict a potential obstacle or distraction you may face while working on the activity.

4. How will you deal with the disruption? Create an "IF-THEN" method for coping with this barrier/distraction. ("IF I come across X, THEN I shall deal with it by performing Y").
5. Follow your step-by-step strategy and "enter the room with a plan" to carry out your desired activity.

Establish Beginning and End of Tasks

Many chores and meetings – such as college courses, job meetings, religious events, television shows, a time-based exercise regimen, and so on – have defined (or at least relatively predictable) start and finish times. Because they are time-bound, these tasks are easy to organize and fit around other obligations in your daily planner.

Many projects do not have such strict time constraints. You may want to perform some housekeeping or write on a paper for a course, but no one will know if you do not complete these duties. It is simple to justify, "I can work on this later."

If you work on it later, it won't be an issue. However, time constraints are a serious issue for individuals with ADHD and anxiety. Many people report putting off work or a task (such as having clean clothes or cleaning up their space) until the last minute.

Tasks with no clear ends are more difficult to plan. You've seen road signs near major cities informing drivers about the expected journey time to different exits and interchanges. Even though there would be a delay, drivers may modify their attitudes and expectations when given a firm time estimate to their destination instead of it being ambiguous. It is the same with tasks placed into the daily planner—it is useful to know when they begin and when they will conclude to modify expectations and encourage follow-through.

Many individuals with ADHD and anxiety claim that they "work best at the last minute," yet those who seek therapy for ADHD frequently experience severe issues (Hallowell, 2022) of this habit of "brinkmanship." Even if you can pull an "all-nighter" or spend long sessions catching up on work or housework (both of which are romanticized as "hyperfocus"), these tactics come at a cost to your physical and mental well-being. Setting end deadlines for projects mitigate the chance of getting into this crisis cycle.

A coping method for open-ended work that uses the daily planner style is to plan realistic start and finish times. Projects like writing a research paper for college, preparing a presentation for work, or cleaning and arranging a space at home may be overwhelming. People may spend many hours on any of these vital chores without accomplishment.

Although these are the chores for which you should set aside time in your daily planner, there will almost certainly never be enough time to perform them all at once. Even if you have a free calendar with no obligations, it is unlikely that you or anybody else would arrange and complete an eight-hour block of time dedicated to "cleaning and organising my bedroom" or "writing the prescribed 20-page paper." You don't spend that much time on things you like, much alone a task or project.

First and foremost, you should intend for the start and finish dates to be reasonable and attainable expectations for work performance, especially those that are not inherently fun or "motivating." Using the previous example, you may not be able to commit to cleaning a room for eight hours, but you will be able to manage 30 minutes. You're still doing a job, but you're reducing your attention and expectations by setting a time limit for a task that is reasonable and allows you to participate in a constructive activity. This coping approach is another step in "breaking down chores" to make them more manageable. Rather than increasing your desire for the activity, try "lowering the bar" and setting a more fair expectation.

A second advantage of having start and finish times is that it makes work scheduling easy, fostering follow-through. These are the chores you should usually put on your daily to-do list. This method is handy when working on a huge project that cannot be finished all at once. You choose a certain section of the project to focus on within a set period, allowing you to make progress without feeling overwhelmed (and then procrastinating).

Finally, using start and finish times for assignments is a good method to manage days when you have a lot of free time, such as a leisure day or a weekend. This free time does not mean that you have to be "productive" all day and plan everything. However, this strategy may assist in identifying certain appropriate duties (including entertainment and downtime) that can serve as anchors throughout the day and prevent the sensation of coming to the conclusion of a "free day" and feeling like it was a waste.

Activities for Self-Care

It is critical to prioritize self-care, including your health and wellness, via activities such as exercise, meditation, hobbies, and relaxation. You may believe that these are "simple" things that take up too much of your time and that you should be focusing on more productive duties.

Yes, you are more prone to put off necessary tasks that are not instantly reinforcing. ADHD, on the other hand, hinders planning as well as following through on personal interests. We do not want you to abandon fun hobbies, but rather be more conscious of how they fit into your day and be proactive in scheduling time for them as a reward for the time spent on other duties. Balancing your energy and effort is part of the rhythm of your timetable.

It is critical to arrange breaks during the day, providing time for meals and exercise, among other things. Because of the attention and poor self-monitoring characteristics of ADHD and anxiety, you may miss indications that you are hungry, tired, or other signs about your present physical condition that influence your performance. Making time for self-care ensures that you pay attention to your well-being.

One impediment to prioritizing self-care is the idea, "I can't think about exercise when I have so much to accomplish" (or "I wasted my time earlier in the day; therefore, I can't justify allowing myself to continue the exercise." We see self-care (and recreational) duties as critical to encouraging the completion of other "work" and "education" tasks, as well as any other significant commitments.

Self-care is crucial to enhancing general well-being and productivity, rather than "wasting time." Of course, there may be occasions when you must sacrifice a self-care action for another goal (for example, "I will have to forego my downtime on the Internet today to be ready for my speech tomorrow."). However, it is generally good to continue self-care activities and not deprive oneself of the benefits that sleep, exercise, and a balanced diet give.

Statements of logic:

- "I'm not going to sit here and let my anxiousness fester." "I'm going to get up and walk around to get rid of this extra adrenaline."
- "I don't have to deal with this right now. Instead, I'm going to burn it off deliberately."
- "I'm committed to keep going ahead and permanently reducing this anxiety!"

When in doubt, take action. Move around and get some exercise. While this is not a long-term solution to this situation, it is something you can do every day to improve your mood and keep you physically fit. Excessive worrying, as well as anticipatory anxiety, are reduced by exercise. Anything that might briefly alleviate our anxiousness is beneficial and is a step in the right direction.

So, remember not to sit motionlessly, dwell, or be afraid. Don't succumb to defeat. Instead, get up, leave, and get going. By getting more active, you may reduce your anticipatory worry.

The Importance of Medication

Many adults with ADHD need medication as part of their therapy. Medicine does not treat ADHD; instead, it alleviates symptoms while active.

Certain neurotransmitters appear to be predominantly and directly affected by medications that most successfully address the primary symptoms of ADHD. The neurotransmitters responsible for this are dopamine and norepinephrine. Both neurotransmitters seem to be involved in ADHD's attentional and behavioral symptoms. A pharmaceutical trial may assist in establishing which treatment works best for each person and at what dose. Typically, the study starts with a low dosage progressively raised at three to seven-day stages until clinical advantages are obtained.

Medication usage reports differ. For some, the benefits are enormous; for others, medicine is beneficial; and for others, the outcomes are small. Attention span, impulsivity, and on-task behavior frequently improve in organized situations. Some adolescents increase their frustration tolerance, cooperation, and even their penmanship. Interactions with families, friends, and educators may improve as well.

Chapter Five: Time and Task Management - Define, Prioritize, and Construct What You Do

You have the essential tools to manage your time, projects, effort, and energy if you have a notion of your complete to-do list, prioritising a daily to-do list, and a daily planner system. You may have created numerous intricate lists and well-designed strategies in the past but did not follow through on them. Thus, how successfully you control your ADHD and anxiety is determined by how well you play the time management game.

This chapter will concentrate on time management "moves" and techniques that will assist you in putting together the many skills and tools we've examined so far to follow through on plans.

Tasks Can be Defined In Specific and Behavioral Terms, This is How to Do It

What is the specific task you are avoiding? What are your first instincts in response to this task? Is there any way to characterise the assignment to encourage completion?

We've spoken about the need to describe a job or activity in as clear and behavioral terms as feasible. On your to-do list or in your daily planner, you may have items such as "work on the yearly update," "clean up the house," "exercise," or "do readings for economics class."

Some people may interpret these brief statements into action plans, such as utilising the plan to "clean up the kitchen" as a trigger to empty the dishwasher. Individuals with ADHD, and anxiety, on the other hand, have difficulty converting these broadly defined activities into a particular sequence of behaviors that encourages follow-through ("There is too much to accomplish. I'm at a loss for words. This is too much for me right now.").

It is helpful to express your goal in particular behavioral phrases or action steps that you may do on your daily to-do list or while carrying out such chores. For more significant projects comprising several more minor activities, such as a monthly report or cleaning up a room, defining a minor component step offers you an attainable aim that keeps you motivated.

To put it another way, you want to "lower the bar" to enhance the chance of getting started.

Working on the yearly report, for instance, might be redefined as "spend 30 minutes analysing the sales figures for the last year" or "use last year's report as a framework to input information for this year." "Cleaning up the house" may mean "removing rugs and furniture to clean." This approach is a variation in breaking down a major work into smaller pieces. Of course, we've all heard this advice and know what we should do, but the key here is to plan out how we'll accomplish it, down to the tiniest initial step that bridges the gap between inactivity and action (Hofmann, 2007).

In contrast, persistent procrastination on a task might indicate that you do not yet have a clear beginning point. The next part focuses on approaches to describe the critical initial step that distinguishes between procrastination and involvement.

Establish The Most Important Tasks for Your To-Do List

After determining your primary commitments and duties for the day; it is critical to align your calendar with your daily to-do list. Activities on your daily to-do list, such as completing a particular errand or committing time to an essential work or school assignment, may be planned in your daily planner.

For instance, you may have a weekly 2 p.m. class noted as an obligation in your daily planner, but you do not need to include it on your daily to-do list. If you are due to give a presentation at the next class meeting, you may designate the break before that session in your planner for final touches, which is an item on the daily to-do list.

The daily planner is similar to Google Maps in that you may begin with a broad view of the overall region and the path you will follow. You may zoom in on increasingly more comprehensive views of particular weeks, days, and segments of a single day, similar to the map function. The daily to-do list becomes the street-level view, in which you get to a task using step-by-step guidance. Of course, as with excellent instructions, having appropriate and correct steps for these activities (Hallowell, 2022), which we will describe next, is essential.

Behavioral Engagement - Start By Defining the Smallest Steps

Despite the above-listed solutions, you may still have trouble getting started on activities. The types of work on which you continue to procrastinate are probably those for which even modest steps are relatively tedious or uncomfortable, such as chores, academic duties (reading textbooks, writing assignments), or administrative responsibilities of adult life (dealing with taxes or finances).

These and other chores elicit unpleasant ideas and sentiments which impede follow-through, even on the first steps. To get started on these activities, describe the simplest actions necessary to begin the activity in rigorous, behavioral phases. These early actions may not include finishing the work, but they are important stages (Hofmann, 2007) that allow you to "touch" a task rather than keep it at arm's length.

This method is intended to assist you in breaking down jobs into their specific behavioral components, similar to a food recipe. "I don't know how to cook," you may remark, or "I can't do it." However, after you follow the listed procedures, you are involved in the job rather than separated from it. It's a beneficial task to see how other activities are broken down into steps. Do it by yourself.

A college attendee, for instance, may have academic tasks for many courses. She schedules 30 minutes for one of the readings, intending to go as far as she can in that time. Despite knowing that it is necessary, she cannot tear himself away from the computer to begin the reading. The initial stage in behavioral engagement is to cease the task interfering with the goal and then take the smallest possible step toward the target task.

For the college student, the objective becomes "get up and go pick up the textbook." The following step is to "open to the first page of the chapter." The next stage is to "read the opening line of the chapter," which the student is now doing. Now, she is no longer delaying the task. She may quit reading after the first phrase or after 12 minutes, or she can read for the whole 30 minutes (and beyond). Whatever occurs next, the student now has an action-based framework for dealing with procrastination rather than merely attempting to "not procrastinate."

"This is so simple, it won't assist me," you may think in response to this coping tip. However, if you are delaying duties, it is clear that something is wrong with your attitude. As an illustration, it may seem silly to have to manage a phone call by defining the first step as "pick up a receiver" or "find the individual in my contact list." Still, most individuals with ADHD have instances of task procrastination that are equally absurd ("I can't believe I still haven't made that phone call. I could have blown my chance."). The first stage of behavioral engagement is to define a job as such an embarrassingly easy action step that failing to complete it becomes silly (Hofmann, 2007).

We invite you to do an experiment where you just observe how you postpone chores throughout your day to discover how you do not complete things. Of course, not all work delays result from procrastination, but the experiment illustrates the process.

It may be anything as basic as not cleaning up a crumpled piece of paper on the floor that had bounced off the edge of a trash can, or it could be something more personal, such as a job assignment or an exercise. The practice requires you to assist yourself in observing the many thoughts, emotions, and escape actions that comprise your procrastination profile. Procrastination is a habit that may become automatic, like tying your shoes.

The capacity to notice the indicators of procrastination as they emerge, on the other hand, helps to make the process less automatic, offers signals that you are postponing work, and opens up multiple intervention opportunities for using your coping methods.

The tactics listed above intend for you to get you to the brink of your preferred action plan. Finally, you must take that first step that signifies truly accomplishing what you set out to achieve. Each of the above phases will assist you in preparing for the work and taking figurative baby steps toward completion rather than instantly sliding into the overlearned habit of procrastination.

It's crucial to realise that you may not be "in the mood" to complete the activity or action. In reality, keep in mind that you may overestimate how little energy and attention are necessary to begin work. The last push to begin a task or activity is analogous to legislative "swing votes"—it does not have to be unanimous; merely reaching a 51–49 outcome is sufficient to initiate behavioral involvement. "Once I got started," most people say, "it wasn't as horrible as I feared."

Breaking a Task or Activity into Steps

Zeno's paradoxes is a philosophical puzzle collection. While attempting to leave a place, you must first reach the halfway point between yourself and the exit. As you go toward the doorway, you will reach a new midway, and each subsequent attempt to depart the area will need you to reach the next midpoint.

The paradox is that you should be unwilling to leave a room since you can endlessly reduce the distance to the exit without ever leaving. When confronted with chores on your daily to-do list, you may often feel like you are attempting to leave the room since it seems as if you can never get things started.

Zeno's paradox demonstrates how most jobs are broken down into ever-smaller component pieces. More significantly, taking the appropriate initial step toward completing a job provides you the confidence that "I can do this."

When laying out your priority duties, you will come across certain jobs that cause you to feel fear, overwhelmed, or as if you can't cope with them. Rather than reflexively ignoring them ("I can't manage this right now!"), the first step is to assess what you want to achieve and if your objective – at least as you presently see it – is too large or imprecise. The general goal remains vital, such as "arrange my room" or "work on paper for school," but it is difficult to see a means to get started in such broad terms.

You may break the major project into its component phases like you would leave a room. Thus, "arrange my room" is divided into three tasks: eliminating clutter that does not belong in the space, selecting what objects will remain in the room, and determining where each kept item belongs.

Even the initial step of decluttering may be too stressful. If such is the case, you can reduce this step to a single item, such as "I will begin by picking up any dishes in my room and taking them to the kitchen." Similarly, a job or school project is divided into phases. Before diving into the monthly report write-up, data may need to be gathered or examined (Hofmann, 2007).

Time spent organising one's ideas or preparing a paper might assist a student to start a project without needing to leap immediately into writing. Even if you have begun your write-up, you may put off returning to the incomplete document. The aim of "continue writing the report" is demanding; therefore, word the first, smaller step toward this goal as "I will read the previous paragraph I wrote and then write the first line of the following paragraph."

The key concepts describe the task in basic and behavioral terms to transform the task goal into an activity you can do. To combat procrastination, you will be able to reduce most projects to the simplest initial step that you feel capable of doing.

A simple method to begin "touching" work and school assignments are to ensure you have accurate information about the task's limits, due date, and so on (e.g., "I will review the syllabus to ensure I am clear about the assignment."). Simply opening a computer file for a work assignment or picking up a textbook to study for a class are basic action steps that dramatically boost the chance of completing the activity.

Time spent imagining and preparing the activity is a little step of involvement and an exposure exercise that improves your capacity to confront something you normally avoid and flee. A spreadsheet, a piece of paper, or index cards may be used to separate the many parts of a huge project, including your starting point, the targeted end point, and all the intermediate phases. This practice is beneficial when a job is vast and has a deadline.

This kind of undertaking necessitates "doing a little bit" each day instead of completing everything at the last minute in a frenzy. Even if you intend to commit an hour or two to an activity, such as housework, errands, or yard maintenance, a strategy for breaking down and arranging your actions is beneficial (which can include a reward). Breaking an activity down into manageable steps is an important method for getting started and staying on track.

Realistic Expectations - This is How to Establish Them

The film Apollo 13 dramatized a human space trip to the Moon in 1970. Due to technical problems, the space trip was aborted mid-flight. The mission's goal shifted from landing on the Moon to returning the men to Earth successfully. The astronauts' damaged spaceship had an insufficient battery capacity to power the various computer systems required to reenter Earth's atmosphere. NASA experts on the ground had to figure out the best way to reactivate these systems while conserving energy and without emptying the batteries (Hallowell, 2022).

Some individuals with ADHD and anxiety prioritize morning exercise (Hofmann, 2007), which allows them to concentrate on high-priority chores first thing in the morning before moving on to other things. Others like to "warm up" with lower-priority administrative activities first thing in the morning before tackling higher-priority, more difficult tasks.

Students learn that some times of the day are preferable to others for focusing on academic duties, such as dedicating mornings to writing projects and afternoons to required readings. Similarly, specific pivot points in the day might be recognized as excellent times for monotonous chores, such as sorting through the mail as soon as you get home from work or trying to catch up on emails for 15 minutes after coming from a lunch break at work.

Understanding "how your brain works" is critical to planning your timetable and honestly judging how well your routine works. Someone else's adaptive warm-up task is another person's escape behavior. The trick is to figure out what is feasible and sustainable for you.

Do not be afraid to make necessary changes

Life is unpredictable. Situations may develop that will need adjusting your expectations and plans, such as skipping work to pick up a sick kid from school or attending an emergency automobile repair. Aside from the technicalities of restructuring your calendar, the daily planner also serves as a coping aid for managing, or at the very least reducing, the emotional stress that comes with unanticipated changes.

Using your planner allows you to see what adjustments you need to make and how to accomplish them. To accomplish a job by a deadline, you may have to compromise, such as missing a gym visit or delaying an appointment. Having a record of your planned obligations, on the other hand, gives a framework for dealing with the issue by taking the required measures to cancel and reschedule appointments, as well as any other modifications that must be made to successfully "handle the problem."

In addition to dealing with an unexpected change in your schedule, the daily planner assists you in determining if the occurrence was unexpected or whether it was the consequence of procrastinating or underestimating the importance of particular chores. These abilities and processes enable you to learn from errors more orderly and reduce their recurrence.

Plans for Implementation

The reality of coping with procrastination is that you will face many distractions and lower-priority chores that are simpler, more pleasurable, or just emerge as handy reasons for flight after your early zeal wears off. It is beneficial to have implementation strategies in place to ensure follow-through.

Implementation intention plans, based on research on children with ADHD, are intended to externalise executive functioning by predicting challenges to your aims and preparing strategies to manage those threats. Consider these tactics to be malware for threats to your time management strategy.

A college student, for example, who expects to study an assigned material for 30 minutes would almost certainly confront several distractions. Even if he's reading at the library, he could see a buddy pass by, get a text message, or have a spontaneous idea about something he wants to do later. Each of these harmless diversions has the potential to throw him off course.

Develop detailed plans for these occurrences as part of the implementation plans. Using if-then plans to build a strategy for starting, such as "If I go to the library, then I will read for at least 30 minutes," or "If I encounter a friend, then I will tell her I have to finish reading but will see her later" are excellent ways to start these detailed plans.

Instead of continuously concentrating on an overarching goal to sustain motivation, implementation plans address particular threats to the current plan (which is part of a bigger aim), compatible with the approach of "entering the room with a plan." Given how readily people with ADHD may be diverted, we focused on establishing these if-then strategies to deal with different task-interfering distractions, transitions between activities, returning after breaks, etc.

There's no assurance you won't get sidetracked or succumb to distraction. Being interested in the activity, thinking through possible distractions, and building your adaptive reactions (including preemptive steps like turning off your phone) all work together to raise the possibility of greater follow-through on your objectives than in the past. Furthermore, these approaches give you steps to engage or reconnect with tasks (Hofmann, 2007).

Escape that Habits Introduction

Regardless of the coping mechanisms discussed above, including implementation tactics, it is important to know the distractions you are subject to while procrastinating. You will develop a list of "usual suspects" of escape behaviors, which may include checking your email, social media usage, or other things that, if not pleasurable, are less stressful than the possibility of your job plans.

It is important to transition from not realizing they procrastinated to acknowledging that they were engaging in escape behavior. These "escape" activities may be exploited as task completion incentives, shifting their behavioral function from negative reinforcement of off-task behavior to positive reinforcement of on-task conduct.

What are the most typical jobs, websites, devices, games, etc.? If you find yourself doing them, are you avoiding something else? Instead of completing a key job, such as cleaning or napping, are there other useful activities you can do instead of completing a key job?

Procrastination is a combination of actions that result in the postponement of duties. To begin rewriting your procrastination "script," you must first comprehend it and unravel the different aspects that put you at risk for this behavior. Another important aspect of combating procrastination is controlling your thoughts about what you set out to do.

Procrastination and its Related Thoughts

Your current attitude toward a task is an important component of the procrastination script. We're talking about the reflexive or instinctive thoughts and emotions you have when faced with a priority task (or any other kind of activity you wish to perform). Each job on your daily to-do list was specified in behavioral terms, sounded attainable, and was a priority when you created it. You were probably more excited about the potential of taking action and your capacity to do so.

However, when confronted with the work, you discover that your perspective has shifted. You begin to believe that you are not up to this right now and that there are so many other annoying jobs you can get done right now; it would be better for you to accomplish them instead of this other duty.

You are suddenly off doing something else, possibly even realising that you are delaying. Later, when you discover you did not stick to your plan and wasted crucial time, you feel bad about yourself, thinking, "I had plenty of time to do this today. Again, how did I do this? I'm not sure when I'll have the opportunity to focus on it in the next few days, and I'm racing the clock. This is terrible!"

The description above is not comments made by you or others but rather descriptions of your current flow of ideas or self-talk. These "automatic ideas" regarding your top priorities happen without your conscious knowledge. You may be unaware of how swiftly and powerfully they impact your emotions and behavior. The concepts felt realistic while bouncing around in your mind but ultimately counterproductive.

Cognitive behavioral therapy's "cognitive" component is how this automatic thinking is managed. Negative or distorted thinking does not correlate with ADHD, but as the case above shows, it does not make living with ADHD any easier. When people without ADHD postpone a task, they experience similar ideas, but they can modify their behaviors to guarantee timely follow-through.

Adults with ADHD, on the other hand, constantly relapse into the same procrastination cycle despite suffering consequences. Capturing and modifying these habitual thoughts is a vital coping skill to master.

The first step in addressing negative automatic thoughts regarding work or goal is to catch them by asking, "What am I thinking right now?" These ideas are sometimes stated in quick phrases rather than grammatically perfect sentences ("Oh no," "I loathe this stuff," a series of expletives, etc.). In truth, procrastination may begin with a true statement ("The gym is packed after work.") However, this might set off a chain of assumptions that lead to procrastination ("I won't be able to locate any available equipment, so I won't be able to complete my exercise. I'm too tired to deal with crowds, so I won't go tonight."). That evening watching TV and eating too many cheese puffs led to self-criticism and irritation with the missed exercise ("I could have gone to the gym. I would have finished by now. Now I have to find time to make up for the lost time.").

It is critical to be conscious of how your ideas cause you to postpone. Automatic thoughts are frequently distorted and influence your sentiments about work. You begin to freak yourself out of completing anything without having a chance to start, increasing the possibility of turning to avoid work via an escape habit.

You must:

1. Determine the specific task that you are putting off.
2. Identify your ideas about completing the work. How do you exaggerate the bad parts of a task?

3. Identify your thoughts regarding the activity, such as boredom or a gut sensation of "ugh, I don't want to do this."
4. Now, consider and emphasise why this work is important to you and how it will feel to do it.
5. Identify the favourable characteristics of your capacity to do the work that you may lessen.
6. Consider how happy you will feel after you have completed the assignment.
7. Regardless of how you feel, break down the work into tiny, initial steps you can do to get started.
8. Allow yourself a few seconds of pain and doubt while taking step #7.
9. You have stopped procrastinating.

Chapter Six: Motivation, Emotions, and Energy

The vast majority of obligations you will encounter in life will necessitate consistent and numerous efforts over time to accomplish or sustain, such as finishing a large project for work, keeping up with school tasks, performing home repairs, or recurring tasks, such as paying bills, preserving an exercise routine, trying to manage household chores, and so on.

"Sometimes I can get started on a goal and stay going for a short while, but I cannot sustain it," many people with ADHD and anxiety remark (Hallowell, 2022), which is a characteristic of the executive dysfunction and motivational deficiencies that underpin ADHD.

While different planning, organisational skills, and other "getting started" skills will continue to be helpful, there are extra measures you can take to keep your plan on track, remain on top of things, and avoid spiraling into chronic and painful procrastination.

Motivation - Produce it!

When dealing with the subject of plan follow-through, the question of motivation often comes up. Many individuals with ADHD and anxiety may strive to attain a goal (exercise) or complete a certain task (test, paying bills) but, despite their best efforts, succumb to an apparent lack of drive. This circumstance reminds us of a comment attributed to the late fitness instructor Jack LaLanne, stating at the age of 93, "I'm feeling terrific, and I still have sex nearly every day." Returning to the executive dysfunction perspective of ADHD, motivation is described as the capacity to develop a feeling about a task that supports follow-through without immediate reward or consequence (and often in the face of some short-term pain).

In other words, motivation is the capacity to make oneself "feel like" executing a job even when there is no compelling reason to do so. Consequently, you'll have to find a method to make yourself want to exercise or prepare for a midterm test that's still a few days away before you get the results you want.

You "know" cognitively that these are wonderful ideas, but bad sentiments (including boredom) or a lack of enthusiasm about a task undermine your efforts to begin. One of the most prevalent cognitive mistakes shown by individuals with ADHD while delaying is the exaggeration of emotional unpleasantness connected with commencing a task, generally accompanied by a reduction in the good sensations associated with it.

Adults with ADHD face the double disadvantage of having more trouble creating positive feelings (motivation) required to participate in activities and having more difficulty resisting the temptation of more immediate distractions, particularly those that give an escape from pain. Individuals with ADHD have frequently had more than their fair share of difficulties and failures in many critical facets of their life from a developmental viewpoint.

In our view, many daily tasks and activities have been connected with a degree of stress and little apparent reward, exacerbating the motivational issues that ADHD individuals already confront.

We will use the metaphor of food poisoning to demonstrate how one's learning history because of ADHD poses (Hallowell, 2022) impedes pursuing important personal objectives. Food poisoning is caused by consuming contaminated food. It is an adaptive reaction in which your brain and digestive system detect the presence of a toxin in your body and respond with nausea and quick evacuation of the toxin by diarrhea, vomiting, or both.

Even after you have completely recovered and determined that you had food poisoning, the sight and smell of the meal, even before it reaches your lips, can revive protective emotions of nausea owing to the past connection of the stimulus (the food) with disease and discomfort. You may make all the rational reasons for your safety and assurances that the meal is safe, but your body will still have this first unpleasant response. To break the food poisoning connection, increasing exposure to unspoiled morsels of the meal is required (often mixing it in with "safe" food in difficult situations).

Similarly, in your attempts to build and maintain excellent habits for controlling ADHD, you will come into certain chores that cause pain while recognizing the importance of the work at hand. As a result, it is critical to generate just enough drive to shift out of avoidance and take a "taste" of the work you are putting off.

You will need to feel like performing the activity you are avoiding, at least enough to take the initial steps toward doing it. Performing the activity does not imply that you must be zealous about what you want to undertake. You simply need to know that you can carry out your immediate action plan, even if you are not "in the mood" to do so.

This kind of motivation is developed by narrowing your attention to the processes required to engage in the desired goal. Starting a task frequently alters your perspective because you deal with the reality of your actions rather than being lost in anticipations and ambivalence.

Furthermore, once you take the initial step toward completing the assignment, you are no longer delayed. Rather than striving to increase your motivation to meet the demands of the activity, you may decrease (Hofmann, 2007) the initial demands of the task to match your existing motivation level and get to the point where you declare, "I can do this."

As described in the preceding chapter, taking little actions to "touch" a task allows you to get started on it without needing to feel motivated—action frequently precedes motivation. Returning to the food poisoning metaphor, these procedures assist you in tasting a little enough piece of the previously hazardous food to enable you to rebuild good associations with it and allow your brain and body to feel secure again. In implementing strategies to manage ADHD better, you may encounter some deeply ingrained avoidance habits that seem immune to change and take more specific effort to overcome.

Energy - Manage it!

Time management entails energy management as well. The explanation for procrastinating is often wrapped up in the remark "I'm not up to this," which reflects the reality that you are fatigued, stressed, or in some other unpleasant condition. You infer that you lack the necessary energy to complete a work, which is likely accompanied by a mistaken explanation for postponing it ("I have to be at my best or else I will be unable to accomplish it.").

Comparable to reframing time, reframing energy might help you respond to the "I'm not up to this" emotion. Thinking through a work's actual behavioral and energy needs provides a more accurate perspective on the original and sometimes skewed rationale. Remember that you simply need "enough" energy to get started. As a result, being "too weary" to empty the dishwasher or do the laundry might be reframed to perceive these duties as taking just a little energy and concentration.

Utilising this kind of reframing to address automatic ideas regarding energy on activities that demand a bit extra pep in the step.

76

For example, it is typical for individuals to be hesitant to exercise because they believe they are "too fatigued to exercise." That assumption may be shifted to reflect the energy necessary for the minor stages in the "exercise script" that serve as the "launch sequence" for going to the gym ("Are you too tired to retrieve your workout clothes? Carry them to the car?" and so on). You may also ask yourself whether you've ever seen somebody slumped over the workout equipment at the gym because they ran out of energy from attempting to push themselves when they were "too weary."

Instead, you may rely on prior experience to know that you will feel better and more invigorated after exercising; you will sleep much better, be more rested, and benefit from sticking to your exercise schedule. At the very least, going through this process rather than succumbing to the want to avoid increases (Hofmann, 2007) the likelihood that you will make a reasoned choice rather than an impulsive one regarding the assignment.

A specific energy management problem essential to sticking to plans is your capacity to sustain energy (and hence effort) over extended periods. Anxiety management is an endurance sport. Good soccer players are known to find their rest on the field to play the whole 90 minutes of a game. Likewise, you must control your speed and effort throughout the day. The rhythm of your daily planner's many chores and duties influences your energy. It is critical to participate in self-care throughout the day, including proper sleep, mealtime, rest, and recreational activities to recharge your batteries.

Even at work, you may follow up a demanding activity – such as working on a project – with more administrative activities – such as replying to emails or phone conversations – that do not take as much mental energy or, at the very least, indicate a transition to a new task. Similarly, you may complete different duties earlier in the evening and spend the remainder of the time resting at home.

A good reminder is that there are methods to make certain jobs manageable, if not joyful, by tying them to favored hobbies for which you have greater drive. Folding clothes while watching the television or performing yard work or domestic duties while listening to music on an iPod, are instances of how you can combine responsibilities and pleasure hobbies. Furthermore, enjoyable experiences and job accomplishments will most likely be satisfying and stimulating.

The Benefits of Reward Systems

The usage of reward systems is another fundamental behavioral concept that can improve motivation and follow-through. The Premack Principle is a well-established psychological concept that states that following the accomplishment of a less wanted job with the reward of an extremely desirable task increases the chance of doing the less desired task. Examples of the idea include eating veggies before dessert and completing schoolwork before watching television.

A pleasant reward acts as a carrot at the end of a stick to incentivize a work that is not intrinsically joyful. The reward should be something you want and, preferably, something you can only have by finishing that activity. For example, you may reward regular exercise with a fruit smoothie or completion of a study session for a final test with a music download.

These behavioral goals are not immutable physical rules. You will be tempted to break them ("I want a smoothie but don't feel like moderate exercise will be an advantage on tomorrow's exercise."). The mere linkage of activity with a reward, on the other hand, will most certainly boost its salience for you. At the very least, it causes a halt in time and action (behavioral suppression) that enables you to think about the job rather than putting it off impulsively.

How to Accept and Retrain Your Emotions

Another aspect of living with ADHD that you should be aware of is that you will most likely have difficulty managing your emotions. This difficulty may not always imply that you suffer from a mood or anxiety issue. Rather, emotional regulation challenges associated with ADHD are characterized by difficulty with emotions in circumstances that most individuals experience, whether unfavourable, such as dealing with job stress, or positive, such as receiving exciting news.

While anybody will have an emotional response to upsetting news – such as a large car repair costs or an unforeseen and inconvenient change in one's work schedule – the individual with ADHD is more likely to overreact, which may cause additional stress. Someone with ADHD may take longer to cool down, later realising their anger was unwarranted but then having to cope with the consequences of the response in addition to the initial cause of stress.

Thus, controlling ADHD necessitates the development of "emotional endurance" for dealing with things that, in the short term, you do not want to accomplish but that, in the long run, are associated with cherished objectives. Again, executive dysfunction makes these undertakings more challenging for those with ADHD. When confronted with duties or events that cause emotional distress, it is critical to realise that the only way out is to follow the event through to the end.

You will often suffer pain when confronted with chores that you normally avoid. A coping skill in these instances is the knowledge that you can identify your emotions, describe them, and yet follow through on the actions needed in the work you want to do, even if you are still uncomfortable.

Our elementary approach to mindful tolerance of emotional pain associated with ADHD management is the capacity to detect emotions, tolerate them, and remain on track with what you are doing. Just as you may have to accomplish something despite a headache, there will be certain things that you can do despite an emotional "pain," which is frequently worrying, boredom, or a sense of "ugh."

One emotional management tactic is to behave in the opposite direction of your present mood, known as the "method acting" approach or behaving "as if." If you are furious about anything, you may make yourself grin or clap your hands together and say loudly, "okay, enough TV, it is time to tackle my report" to get started on a job.

Merging these skills with other task engagement methods – like defining the first step and setting reasonable time expectations – helps you respond to the task and changes your relationship with these emotions to tolerate them rather than eliminating them as a precondition to starting the task.

As you begin to face tasks that you have previously avoided, you will discover that you are better able to do so without being distracted by your emotions. You will still have sentiments about specific chores, but they will be less likely to throw you off course, offering new and lucrative opportunities for you.

You must:

1. Recognize your emotional responses that lead to your avoidance of an urgent duty.
2. Recognize your sensations, such as boredom, slight anticipation, or "Ugh" ("I don't want to do this right now.")
3. Place your "discomfort" on a scale. How powerful is it? Rate it on a scale of 0 (relaxed) to 10 (worst agony I've ever felt).
4. Notice your feeling and how it feels without attempting to suppress it.

5. Concentrate on breathing slowly and steadily through your emotions.
6. Recognize that your emotions do not have to control your actions.
7. Consider that you can carry out your ambitions while feeling some difficulty.
8. Participate in and concentrate on the lowest behavioral stage for your job.
9. Pay attention to what happens to your emotions after you begin working on the activity.
10. Put these abilities to use in different situations and jobs throughout the day.

Emotional Management in Interactions

In addition to empathy abilities, having a game plan for dealing with emotions generated in these situations is beneficial. There are things you can "do" in these circumstances to effectively manage them, similar to our advice to "make chores manual" to encourage follow through. To begin, determine your "role" or task in the circumstance.

For instance, your position may be "I am an employee listening to what my employer has to say" or "I will be a spouse listening to my wife's views." Classifying your role in an encounter aids in the development of a behavioral script that you may follow, including how you manage your emotions.

Whatever position you play in a circumstance, exposure to distressing information is always a threat. As a result, the second step is to remind oneself to be a good listener and refrain from interrupting the speaker.

It is often beneficial to concentrate on your breathing and keep your muscles relaxed, such as by letting your arms drop freely at your sides. Throughout the encounter, employ empathetic actions and remarks to assist you in concentrating on the task at hand.

Lastly, you will need some time away from the scene following the contact to reflect on what you heard. Even when confronted with a difficult circumstance, things frequently look much more rational and controllable after a few minutes of absorbing them (however, ADHD-related emotion regulation may undermine this viewpoint). You may then return to your "role" description to decide on your plan of action based on the input (for example, "My employer expects me to be on time or I will be written up. Allow me to devise a fresh strategy for getting to work on time.").

Furthermore, after the first wave of emotion has passed, you will most likely have a better perspective on the topic and will be able to detect favourable input you may have gotten but ignored.

The way you approach an encounter has a significant impact on the result. Being able to hear someone out demonstrates your dedication to them. The purpose of developing empathy skills is to remain involved in a dialogue in a productive, in-the-moment way and accept and manage critique. Informing someone that they're correct makes their fury tough to increase.

Because dealing with criticism from others may be a sensitive place for individuals with ADHD, we have presented several communication and empathy techniques. However, you may use the same coping skills to provide feedback to others, bring up sensitive problems, or ask for assistance. For example, if your husband often changes the basket at the front entrance that you use to keep a record of your keys and cell phone so you don't miss them, you will feel adaptive and informative anger.

Chapter Seven: Attitudes, Beliefs, and Self Esteem - Live Your Best Life with ADHD

Adults with ADHD have frequently suffered more failures and frustrations connected with ADHD symptoms, sometimes without understanding the effect of ADHD on them. When you consider a history of poor grades, forgetting or failing to keep commitments to others, and repetitive exhortations about your untapped potential with the need to work much harder, you may develop a negative self-view.

The long-term effect of these frequent setbacks might be the loss of your sense of self, sometimes known as poor self-esteem. These ingrained, long-lasting self-views, or "basic assumptions" about who you are, are seen as a lens through which you perceive yourself, the world, and your role. Therefore, self-esteem and improving it are the focus of this chapter.

Severe adverse experiences linked with ADHD may unjustly skew your vision, leading to a distorted pessimistic perspective of oneself in specific settings. When confronted with experiences that trigger these negative beliefs in the present, you feel powerful emotions, negative thoughts, and a propensity to engage in self-defeating activities, most often resignation and flight.

These basic beliefs may engage some individuals with ADHD in restricted, particular settings; for others, these beliefs impact one's view in most scenarios. It should be noted that, while feeling perplexed by their symptoms in many locations, many individuals with ADHD have an excellent self-view, even though numerous events temporarily upset their confidence.

Catching and Changing Your Automatic Thoughts

Our ideas, which include pictures, emotions, norms, and firmly held beliefs, assist us in categorising and making sense of our experiences. We all have a flow of ideas or interpretations of experiences that happen without awareness but can readily recognize when we pay close attention.

Most of these ideas will be neutral and fleeting, with a more excellent positive-to-negative ratio preferred. The essential point is that these reflexive, automatic thoughts are ripe for distortion, which will interfere with your job completion and usage of coping methods.

Automatic thoughts are distorted thoughts, but they are not illusions; rather, they are inaccurate or impulsive judgments about an occurrence in the absence of convincing proof ("I forgot to contact my friend. She must be upset with me."), or that results from a skewed perception ("I got a bad grade on my essay because the teacher dislikes me."). The meaning in each of these situations is reasonable and probable, but the ultimate conclusion cannot be proven, at least not yet.

On the other hand, a distorted thought may trigger subsequent negative thoughts, resulting in a cascade of assumptions, emotions, and actions that launch a self-defeating episode, such as believing that an instructor does not like you, so you will not get a good grade. Because the instructor does not like you, there is no point in attending class.

Because most erroneous ideas negatively tilt events, Cognitive Behavioral Therapy is also referred to as "positive thinking power."

However, skewed optimistic beliefs, or what is known as the optimistic illusory bias, may occur in ADHD.

Gambling addicts, for example, are extraordinarily optimistic thinkers, even though their predictions contradict all we know about statistical probability. Recording your spontaneous thoughts is to practice understanding your responses to a situation and how they impact your view, mood, and perceived alternatives for action.

The first step in altering your attitude is just paying attention to your natural thoughts. Being able to stop and examine a situation rather than instinctively responding to it is a basic but crucial ability that indicates a method to practice impulse control.

A simple method to practice detecting these ideas is to pay attention when you have an emotional response to anything in your everyday life, no matter how powerful or mild the reaction, especially when you feel yourself delaying. You may have a visible emotional response to a stressor, but you should note your perception of the scenario and how it may be skewed.

You must:

1. Changes in your sentiments, such as discomfort with a task or the fact that you are avoiding a task, are indicators that you are experiencing negative automatic thoughts.
2. Reflect on the setting, task, or event that generated this emotion.
3. What were your thoughts or interpretations?
4. How does this notion affect your emotions and behavior?
5. Do you make any mistakes in your thinking? What new perspectives may you have?

Commitment and Values

Cognitive techniques, like the tactics for producing motivation outlined above, are vital for maintaining your passion for and dedication to longer-term undertakings. It is too simple to indulge in rationalizations and avoidance tactics to avoid a tough job.

Coping drift may occur after you have made a strong start, such as sifting through your daily mail for many weeks or utilising your daily planner, allowing little deviations from your goals to seep in. What begins as solitary, little deviations from your goals, such as "I'm sleepy now. "I'll take care of this later" leads to you reverting to old behaviors and encountering similar problems, such as paying a late charge for overdue payments.

It is a good exercise to review your reasoning and motives for your coping strategies. If you see your coping patterns slipping, the following questions can assist boost the chance of sticking to a specified plan:

- What aspect of this task do I believe I am incapable of completing?
- Have I ever completed an assignment like this before?
- Do I have to be in a good mood to do this?
- Can I focus on the job for five minutes? What would it be like to achieve progress?
- What pleasant experiences may I have?
- How would it feel to begin this work rather than ignore it?
- How difficult will this assignment truly be? Is it something I can handle?
- Is it okay to do this work only to "cross it off my list"?

In addition to these cognitive tactics for re-establishing commitment, remember what you genuinely value about the activity.

The answers to the questions written below might help you nurture and strengthen your dedication to the task:

- What is the significance of this assignment to me?
- How does this activity fit into the bigger picture?
- How far have I progressed toward my final goal? What will be the next step?
- Am I willing to commit to this phase of the plan, even if it is difficult first?
- How will I feel after I finish the task? Will it still seem difficult?
- What are the advantages of beginning this work for me? What are the consequences of procrastination?
- How will it make me feel that I can tackle and complete a challenge like this?
- Can I perform anything relevant to this assignment to know I didn't dodge it?

Change Your Attitude

Human negativity bias indicates that humans are programmed to pay greater attention to frightening and terrifying information than good, reassuring information. This bias may be traced back to when early humans sought food, shelter, and water. Humans were always in a fight-or-flight state because of the continual danger of assault, which promotes anxiety.

Anxiety is a physiological reaction when your body creates a lot of adrenaline and enters danger detection mode. While the worry may overestimate danger, the body attempts to keep you safe.

On the other hand, optimism lowers anxiety in individuals with ADHD. Positive thinking, sentiments of hope, goal-directed action, and confidence are all components of optimism. It's not always about seeing the world through rose-colored glasses.

It's all about how you explain what happens to you in your life, particularly the bad stuff, and what you anticipate to happen in the future. This optimism is how you could change your attitude:

1. Change your brain

Our patterns of thinking are neurologically established. It takes time to develop new pathways in our thinking about ourselves, others, and the world.

The brain is very flexible, adaptable, and changing, with the potential to build new connections across sections of the brain that don't interact very well. It takes time, practice, and fresh experiences to help cement new ideas that we are attempting to practice. The orbitofrontal cortex is a portion of the brain critical for incorporating knowledge from the intellectual, logical, and emotional centers and is larger and better developed in individuals who are more optimistic and less worried. You must comprehend that there are several ways of thinking. Then you must think and determine which patterns of thought are troublesome.

For example, by asking a series of questions, you may learn what was going through their minds when the setback occurred and what they thought about it. Then you can figure out how many of your ideas you're utilising to forecast what will occur in the future and what activities you take or don't take.

The most critical factor is to practice new ways of thinking. Many individuals discontinue their efforts before seeing any sustained and occurred change. After doing a lot of thought editing/active therapy, you will spend time modeling the change of mindset and solidifying or storing those thoughts, so they are more accessible to you.

2. Break down your fears

People with ADHD who are also anxious are likely to have catastrophic thinking, which entails anticipating things to go wrong.They may be tense and find it difficult to relax. They over plan, over worry, and overthink everything. This anxiety is known as a confidence crisis.

Recognizing your fear and learning about it are the antidotes to fear. Understanding the chances of something occurring might help you put your fears into perspective. Many individuals have a mistaken view of the danger that exists in the world. You should remember that 'yes' things may happen, but so can other things. You want to appropriately appraise the possibility of a bad occurrence and your capacity to manage it. Consider a recent distressing occurrence and rate the following on a scale of 0 to 10:

- What are the chances that this will never be resolved or changed?

This book pushes those who tend to exaggerate the chance of something happening to recognize that most situations do resolve themselves over time.

- What are the chances that this occurrence will impact everything in your life?

Considering how the occurrence affects certain areas but not others might help one understand that it isn't as disastrous as first assumed.

- What additional circumstances may have contributed to the occurrence?

It is critical to take ownership of the event's result. Accepting that fear is not the adversary is also a component of this process. There is danger in everything we undertake, and worry exaggerates that risk.

For instance, if you're afraid of making a fool of yourself at school or work, he suggests considering what would happen if that happened and alternative possible outcomes. Is it feasible to speak and have others enjoy what you say? You want to be able to anticipate great possibilities while still understanding that poor results will not kill you.

3. State a positive intention every day

Getting out of bed every morning and saying or writing down your objective for the day will help you get into a good frame of mind. Another option to start the day on a good note is to keep a thankful notebook.

When you get up, think about what you value and adjust your mindset from 'I have to' to 'I get to.' For example, instead of expressing, "I have to take my kids to school," try to say, "I have healthy children who are well enough to go to school," or "I have a vehicle to drive my kids to school."

4. Smile more

Sometimes, a smile is the cause of pleasure, and sometimes joy is the cause of a smile. Occasionally we're pleased; therefore, we smile, but sometimes the reverse is true. You may occasionally mislead your body into feeling pleased by smiling.

It is worth noting that biological, mental, and social factors all contribute to anxiety. Mind-body research increasingly demonstrates that thinking stronger affects how the body functions physically.Parts of the brain that govern emotion or may lead to the fight-or-flight reaction, an anxiety reaction that causes strong hormonal effects on the body and impacts several systems, may begin to harm your health.

People who are too worried and under-relaxed, for example, are more likely to get ill. It's why things like exercise and medicine may assist with anxiety and mood regulation, even if they don't directly address what you're thinking — they sort of bypass that and go right to biology. Positive psychology, as well as mindset science, are making strides. Mind-body therapy examines our expectations since what we feel is likely to happen is more likely to occur.

5. Be mindful

Stop and smell the flowers when you're feeling nervous. Being in tune with nature and present through seeing, experiencing, hearing, and inhaling might change your perspective. There is no anxiety if you can be present in the now since anxiety is something that has occurred or will happen.

Simple Exercises to Raise Your Self Esteem

The activities below will assist you in seeing more of the good aspects of yourself and your life. They are designed to immediately increase your self-awareness so that you may enjoy the positive aspects of your life. We have detailed each activity and then discussed why it will help you boost your self-esteem:

- Make a list of ten things you like about yourself.

It is difficult to notice your great qualities when you have a negative attitude. In truth, no one is entirely good or evil. This activity challenges you to search out your good characteristics to enhance your self-image actively. When you're listing them, make a small comment for each one, detailing what you like about it.

- Continue if you identify more than ten traits.

When you consider love, you may envision the sort of romantic love seen in Hollywood films. That portrayal of love is not only ridiculous, but it is also not where your ideas of love should begin. Your first love should be yourself since you will not be able to love others until you can love yourself because you can't offer what you don't have.

Self-esteem is a healthy habit of loving yourself. You are a one-of-a-kind and amazing human being with a lot to give the world. You must take the time to recognize this.

The Crucial Point

When I was younger, I was taught that loving oneself was a horrible idea. That is not only false but loving oneself is necessary for a happy and healthy existence. Loving yourself is the easiest and fastest technique to boost your self-esteem.

- List your top ten abilities or skills

Recognising your numerous abilities enables you to recognize how much value and worth you have to give others. Write a short remark for each talent indicating how others could benefit or have benefited from it. Continue if you discover more than ten skills. This basic practice is so effective because it causes you to examine your skill set from a viewpoint you are not presently considering.

When you consider your talents, you are most likely doing so from a position of scarcity. This may be beneficial since it allows you to discover talents that you need to improve. By honing these talents, you may enhance your results in both your professional and personal life. However, if you just evaluate the talents you lack, you will miss out on how immensely skilled you are. You must retain a record of your abilities and characteristics as this guarantees that you have a fair picture of your abilities and will raise your self-esteem.

The Crucial Point

There is no reason for you to pretend to be more competent and talented than you are. All you have to do is recognize the talents and qualities you have acquired throughout time. This recognition will help you recognize how awesome you are and will boost your self-esteem for those moments when you need to take a risk and believe in yourself to learn, grow, and improve.

- List five accomplishments that make you proud.

It is easy to lose sight of your past accomplishments when surrounded by negativity. Recognizing prior accomplishments allows you to see that you can do more in the future. Make a full report of each accomplishment. If you go beyond five, keep going until you run out of ideas. Life is a never-ending journey, a never-ending growth. You will often face difficulties that you have never faced before. You have two options for dealing with these challenges:

1. You may either believe that you are incapable of overcoming this new difficulty and so take a step back, or you can take a stride forward.
2. You recognize that you have conquered numerous problems in the past and can do it again.
3. You can't be confident that you'll succeed, but you also can't be positive that you won't. So, my thesis is that it is preferable to trust oneself and accept the challenge. Give it all you've got. Here is where self-esteem comes into play.

To have the requisite self-esteem, you must recognize that you have conquered significant problems in the past. You may boost your self-esteem by documenting and reflecting on your prior accomplishments. Most of the time, self-belief comes from understanding that you have accomplished remarkable things in the past. You have accomplished incredible things in your life; you just need to take the time to acknowledge them (Hofmann, 2007).

The Crucial Point

Again, this isn't about pretending to be someone you're not, as that would never work. Most individuals downplay their accomplishments while exaggerating their misfortunes. You only need to redress the balance by properly recognizing your many accomplishments.

- Describe three times when you overcame hardship.

Realising that you have the strength to deal with whatever life throws at you is one of the most important components of self-esteem. You may see that you can deal with challenging circumstances because of your previous successes in conquering hardship. Write a thorough narrative of the hardship you experienced and the abilities and traits you utilized to overcome it for each instance.

- Remember that you are not required to stop at three.

In life, resilience is crucial. You must believe in your ability to accept and recover from adversity. The most resilient individuals will shrug it off when life throws adversity. They just recognize what needs to be done to get back on track and take the appropriate steps. All who lack resilience feel overwhelmed during difficult circumstances, and stress develops quickly because issues often linger for a long time.

Everyone can be resilient. Some individuals may not believe it since they cannot recollect earlier hardships they have conquered. Recognizing the challenges you've faced can build your resilience and enhance your self-esteem.

The Crucial Point

The confidence that you can overcome hardship is often the most critical aspect. This conviction stems from knowing that you have conquered adversity in the past. Everyone has conquered adversity in their lives; all you have to do is recall those instances.

- Name five people who have aided you.

Do not just name the five individuals; instead, offer a thorough narrative of how they assisted you. This thoroughness lets you realize that other people appreciate you and perceive your worth, and that is why they are eager to help you.

- Continue counting if you have more than five.

The sense that others do not value you weighs heavily on your self-esteem. It is easy to lose trust when you believe you are alone and must handle life's issues independently. But the ancient adage "no man is an island" has a lot of truth. You will only ever be alone in this world if you want to be. Even yet, it is difficult to avoid any human interaction. There will always be those willing to assist you when you need it. All you have to do is reach out to the right folks.

Recording all of the assistance you have gotten from others can boost your self-esteem since it will help you realise that you are not facing any challenges alone. You will know that you may ask for assistance and that, along with others who assist, you will be in a far better position to face any problem.

The Crucial Point

Receiving assistance from others when you are in need will always boost your self-esteem as it will convince you that you are a valuable person. Even if it occurred in the past, remembering occasions when people assisted you can boost your self-esteem.

- Name five people you've helped.

When you have poor self-esteem, you may believe that you are unimportant to others. This practice will help you realise that you have much more to contribute than before. Highlight how you assisted each individual and how they benefited from your assistance.

Don't stop at five if you have more of them.

It's easy to believe you have nothing valuable to give the world, yet this couldn't be farther from reality. Every day, you assist others. Sometimes the assistance you provide is substantial, but it can be tiny, yet it makes the other person's life a bit better and easier.

Consider the small ways people assist you and how much you value that assistance when you get it. That is how people react when you help them. The fact that you can assist others proves that you have something valuable to contribute. Take a minute to notice each time you assist someone else, and it will help boost your self-esteem.

The Crucial Point

Don't believe that to be valuable to others, you must make one enormous contribution to the world. People who make significant contributions to the world are admirable, but the small contributions and gestures given daily make the world run. So, recognize your worth and allow it to boost your self-esteem.

- Make a list of 50 positive aspects of your life.

Many individuals get gratitude and appreciation mixed up. Gratitude is just expressing gratitude to the other person for their assistance. Taking the time to appreciate means understanding how you benefited from your assistance. When you take the time to appreciate, you realize how lucky you are and see your life more positively.

As an example of gratitude, after a pleasant lunch at a restaurant, you may remark to your waiter that you appreciated their service. It may seem easy, but taking a moment to appreciate the advantage you got registers better with your brain than a quick thank you.

One of the most important things to grasp about expressing your gratitude is that it benefits both parties. By expressing your gratitude, you help the other person feel appreciated and realise how fortunate you are to have had a good experience.

The Crucial Point

You may not always have to show your gratitude to others, but continuously taking the time to appreciate the advantages you get can significantly boost your self-esteem. It would benefit both of you if you had the opportunity to show your thanks to others (Hallowell, 2022).

Although 50 may seem to be a large number, the goal here is to get you into the habit of enjoying it. And you may be shocked, but once you start discovering things to be grateful for, you'll want to keep going.

Chapter Eight: Social Skills - Improve Conversations, Friendships, and Fulfill Relationships Without Giving Up Who You Are

People with ADHD often report difficulties in social relationships, whether friendships, romantic relationships, business relationships, or familial relationships. It may be challenging to negotiate social interactions with those they know well, close friends, and strangers.

Most young adults build and develop social ties in their local surroundings, such as at school or college. Nevertheless, young individuals with ADHD prefer to form connections in their immediate surroundings, such as via parental associates or hanging out with friends. This may represent a desire for people to tap into more major social networks and, on occasion, establish friends with peers who are removed from school or are unemployed.

Individuals with ADHD must understand that showing themselves to others influences how others engage with them. This includes how individuals communicate with people and express themselves (verbal communication), their nonverbal posture and motions (body language), and the overall image they project (emotional expressions, ADHD features). This also entails developing social awareness and investigating the impact that any or all of these behaviors have on affecting other people's perspectives.

For instance, inattention to another person may misunderstand ADHD as a lack of interest in what the individual is saying. Adults with ADHD may also be viewed as erratic because they jump from one person to the next or from one subject of discussion to the next. Individuals with ADHD may be prone to making rash judgments and leaping to conclusions due to their impulsivity.

As a result, individuals may accept things at face value based on initial impressions and stereotypical influences. For example, if an acquaintance goes down a hallway without acknowledging them, they may quickly conclude that person does not like them and act in a manner that reflects this, resulting in a self-fulfilled prophecy (Hofmann, 2007). They may fail to consider other possibilities for the lack of recognition, such as the person being in a hurry and concerned with an important subject.

When working to develop your social skills, you must engage in the process correctly. Many individuals fail to enhance their social skills not because they face enormous hurdles but because they approach the work incorrectly and get frustrated. You'll make greater progress if you have the correct mindset, expectations, and attitude to improve.

This chapter discusses certain topics you should know before working on your problems. This chapter addresses some typical issues and concerns regarding developing one's social abilities.

Determine which traits and skills to work on and which to leave alone.

You don't have to alter everything about yourself to improve your social life. Of course, you'll want to address obvious issues that most people would like to avoid, such as shyness and nervousness, poor self-confidence, sloppy communication skills, and a lack of understanding of making friends. Nobody is socially perfect. They can still get by as long as they offer enough positives. If you come across any advice in this book that you disagree with, ask yourself, "Would skipping this tip make me happier overall?" Could I handle the penalties of failing to comply?"

For instance, maybe you're okay with having a franker communication style and also can deal with the reality that it will sometimes irritate certain individuals. Maybe you'll conclude you don't mind being moderately shy, even if it is officially an "issue."

Determine what works best for you

When you consider the pros and drawbacks of a situation, you may decide that you should follow particular social traditions. For example, you'd never give fashion a second thought in your ideal world, but you understand other people do, so you learn to dress a bit better. Or you like spending a lot of time alone, but you force yourself to be around others a little more than you'd like to practice your interpersonal skills and spend time with your friends.

You must determine where you stand and whether or not you are ready to compromise. Changing is not an option if something contradicts your core principles or you just despise it. The practical method might work if you are apathetic about something, and it does not need much effort to accept it. However, there will always be aspects of the social environment in which you will be unable to participate, even if you recognize that it would be sensible. Most individuals will not abandon their religious or political beliefs to fit in.

For example, some men don't like sports but realise they'd have an easier time connecting with others if they did. Some people never grow to enjoy sports, but they can keep up with enough game outcomes and transactions to keep their discussions going. Others can't bring themselves to do even that, and they're content with the tiny inconveniences.

Keep your mind open

Although you don't have to entirely alter or sell yourself out to improve your social life, you should strive to retain an open mind. Be open to new experiences and the chance that you may acquire characteristics or grow to like things you never believed you would love one day.

People change during their life. It's crucial to be loyal to yourself, but not so much that you get stuck in your ways and reject everything new with "No, that's not who I am." Assume you've never danced before, and a buddy invites you to a beginner tango lesson.

Even if you suspect you won't get much out of it, it's too rigid to declare, "No, that's not me!" I don't enjoy dancing and will never like it!" You don't have to try everything that everyone advises, but you never know—you could like partner dancing and not realise it yet.

You can have a satisfying social life without flawless social skills

Many people have enjoyable social lives despite being a little timid and anxious, stumbling in their interactions, not having a lot of exciting interests, or having a few annoying personality flaws. Even the most charming individuals crack poor jokes or have their invitations declined. You don't have to master every ability in this book 100% of the time, and you don't have to win the approval of everyone on the earth.

You only need to be competent enough to get by and have people who accept you for who you are. You don't need every encounter to go perfectly. You simply need enough of them to go well to fulfill your social objectives (for example, if you ask ten people to hang out and only three respond, but they go on to become excellent friends, that's a success).

Improving your social abilities with practice

Social skills are much like any other talent. Reading tips may help you figure out what you need to focus on and make the learning process easier, but you still need to practice to get it down fully. You've spent fewer hours socializing than many of your friends, and you'll need to make up for the lost time.

That may seem apparent, yet some individuals believe social skills are acquired all at once by using the appropriate trick, insight, psychological "hack," or confidence booster when it comes to interpersonal skills. They probably believe this since social skills are non-physical and routine. People intuitively recognize that learning complicated physical talents such as skiing or sketching takes time. Their mind process is, "It's just chatting when it comes to socializing. That is something I am already familiar with. So just give me some secret super-effective conversation formulae, and I'll be all set."

Furthermore, most individuals have discovered that it is simpler to navigate a social setting when they are momentarily more confident than normal. So, there must be a method to be overconfident all of the time. However, although it is possible to feel extraordinarily confident for a short period of time, there is no way to summon that sensation or keep it for the rest of your life. There aren't any shortcuts. They'd be well known if there were, and this book wouldn't be necessary.

Understanding what you are working on as you exercise your social skills

As you practice socializing, you will improve your general talents. You'll use just a few of them in certain situations, while others will demand you to juggle numerous at once.

1. Your quick-thinking capacity. When it's your moment to speak, you can't take long to formulate your answer. Aside from the somewhat predictable initial minute or two. It's impossible to think out what you're going t or how you'll handle every event ahead of time. The best you can do is study some broad rules and hone your improvisational skills.

2. Your multitasking abilities. When communicating with someone, you must constantly pay attention to many things at once. The other person continuously gives signals via their words, actions, and nonverbal communication. You must take it all in, assess, and determine how to respond to your findings on the fly ("They just mentioned they're not acquainted with cycling. I'll have to change the way I deliver my tale."). Simultaneously, you must regulate the signals ("I'm wondering what time it is, but I won't check my watch now since it may make me seem uninterested in their narrative."). As you get more adept at socializing, taking in all of that information and selecting what to do with it becomes less daunting.

3. Your ability to do a range of specific sub-skills such as listening, exerting yourself, or framing an invitation. When you listen carefully, express yourself, or give an invitation, you'll be sloppy and dramatic at first. Still, with practice, you'll acquire a deeper touch and be able to adapt your conduct to the scenario at hand. For example, when you're initially learning how to listen, you can come off as an over-the-top

therapist. With further experience, you'll be able to demonstrate your concern and attentiveness more subtly.

4. Your degree of comfort with several subskills, such as creating eye contact and initiating discussions. Like establishing eye contact or starting a conversation, some subskills can seem awkward or strange at first, but the more you practice them, the more natural they will feel.

5. Your overall understanding of people, what makes them move, and how they respond to certain situations. Everyone is unique, but with enough social experience, you'll begin to recognize broad trends that you may act on. For example, you may observe that individuals who like a certain pastime have similar political opinions and communication styles, and you may modify them appropriately.

6. Your understanding of different social situations and how to manage them. This understanding may be learned by direct experience or by watching those more socially skilled than you. It is easy to get guidance on typical situations, such as how to greet people at a party or decline an outrageous request. Still, you will encounter other scenarios that are too uncommon and obscure to end up in any book in your daily life. When you encounter these unexpected circumstances, you may not always manage them precisely, but you may develop an overall understanding of how to approach them over time.

7. Your understanding of the unwritten social standards of your specific culture, subculture, or group of friends and how to modify basic communication-skills principles to meet them. These unwritten social standards are another reason it is hard to anticipate how to handle every scenario. What is a pleasant conversation style in one culture or among one group of friends may be deemed irritating in another. The only way to

understand the laws of your social environment is to immerse yourself in them and notice them for yourself.

8. Positive attitudes about socializing. A well-meaning but useless kind of social advice proposes adopting beneficial but easier-said-than-done mindsets such as, "Don't care too much about people's perceptions of you" or "Just go out to have fun and don't worry about how well you socialize." It's terrific if you can think like this, but you don't get such worldviews simply by reading about them. Instead, as you mingle more, you'll have numerous tiny achievements and experiences that demonstrate that these are healthy ways to think, and you'll gradually incorporate them into your worldview.

9. Your own social style. There are broad principles for what constitutes a good or bad encounter, but no one correct method to socialize. Everyone has their personality and their own set of talents and shortcomings. There are generally many approaches to each scenario. What works wonderfully for someone else may not work for you at all. Your buddy may be skilled at cheering folks up by listening well. You could be better at making them laugh and distracting them from their troubles.

Methods for Practising Socialization

There are three methods to practice your social skills. If you believe you are socially inexperienced, you may just discover methods to spend more time socializing. This technique is unstructured, but you will still learn new things and refine a range of talents due to the additional hours you will put in. You can

- Increase your socialization with individuals you already know (existing friends, colleagues, classmates, housemates, and family members).

- Find a job that requires a lot of connection with people (such as retail, restaurant waiter, bartender, call center, or sales).
- Sign up for a socializing volunteer role (fundraising, chatting to the elderly, or assisting at a festival).
- Participate in a club, team, or organization.
- Attend online-organized meetings
- Utilize realistic chances for quick, polite conversations with individuals expected to be cheerful and converse with you, such as shop clerks and restaurant waiters.
- Go to a place where individuals may come alone and socialize with other customers (for example, a board game café, a bar, or a pool hall).
- Engage with others online (for example, chatting with people while playing a multiplayer game). Of course, this cannot be a total replacement for face-to-face practice, but it should not be rejected altogether; instead, if travel is a viable possibility, stay in busy, sociable hostels.

A second strategy is to practice a purposeful, organized manner, particularly useful when working on certain talents. If you have problems beginning conversations, you might attend one online-organized meet-up each week and chat with at least five new individuals each time.

If you're having problems with a certain form of encounter, such as asking someone out or saying no to an excessive request, you may practice with a friend or family member. Some organizations, including counseling agencies, provide social skills training groups that allow participants to practice in a safe and supportive atmosphere.

The third option for social practice is to enroll in a class to master performance-oriented interpersonal skills such as public speaking, acting, improv, or stand-up comedy. However, these highly specialized talents may not often translate well into everyday circumstances. A practiced, memorized speech is not the same as a casual, unscripted discussion. Nonetheless, they provide several advantages. Speech training, for example, may teach you how to project your voice and employ confident body language. Taking part in a play may help you overcome your anxiety and dread of being put on the spot. Improv encourages you to be more relaxed, fun, and spontaneous in your interactions. Many individuals feel that knowing they're getting the hang of a scarier ability, such as public speaking, gives them a tiny confidence boost in their regular contacts.

You don't need to spend a lot of time in public chatting to strangers to improve your social skills. Some individuals believe they must engage in casual conversation with strangers at the mall or grocery store. It's one thing to attempt to become accustomed to the beginning and carry on conversations with individuals you don't know.

Talking to strangers is frequently too unpleasant and ineffective if you want to gain social experience in general. Practicing with individuals you already know and are relatively comfortable with rather than strangers you meet in more organized environments such as an art class is preferable.

Getting a Basic Feel for Conversations

Conversations need effort. Even those who are naturally extroverted and seem to be able to speak to anybody become tongue-tied from time to time. So you're not alone if you don't feel comfortable striking up a discussion. Conversations are when the skill aspect of "social skills" truly comes into play since they need you to think on the fly. Three things influence how successfully your encounters go:

- How comfortable and confident you are in them.

- Your technical conversational abilities.
- Your general personality, interests, values, and points of view.

When individuals struggle to strike up a conversation, one of their most common complaints is that they "don't know what to speak about" or "always run out of things to say." This section provides general tips for keeping your interactions continuing.

Determine your conversational objectives.

If you put the typical person in the cockpit of a fighter aircraft and instructed them to go through the start-up procedure and take off as soon as possible, they'd sit there dumbfounded because they wouldn't know where to begin. For the same reason, some individuals become blank during chats.

They find themselves conversing with someone and are aware that they must "make nice conversation," but they are unsure what to do next. It's simpler to speak to people if you have a general notion of where you want to take the conversation. If you feel yourself going blank, you may immediately remind yourself of one of the objectives, which should help you come up with something to say:

Day-to-day socializing objectives

Goal #1: Have a positive engagement for everyone involved.

Goal #2: Learn about the other person and attempt to discover common ground.

Goal #3: Tell the other person something about yourself.

Goal #4: Show you're a friendly person with social skills

Examples

- If you already know the individual, catch up on what you've been up to since your previous meeting (for example, happenings in your life, fun or engaging activities you've done, current issues on your mind).
- If you run into a colleague in the break room, have a quick, polite chat to demonstrate that you're a friendly person who works well with others.
- Before the book club meeting, discuss a subject dictated by the environment, such as what else you've been reading.

Make a general approach to creating conversation.

Good conversationalists often use the tactics listed below. You may use the same tactics more purposefully. A comprehensive game plan may assist since it simplifies and explains what you need to think about, gives confidence that you're utilizing a system that works, and provides some solid, uncomplicated beginning material for practice.

It's a good idea to have many techniques ready to go so that if one fails, you may try another. You may also flip between broad methods as a discussion progresses. You do not have to use the same method for every individual or scenario.

One technique to offer yourself some direction is to inquire about their interests ("I'm going to ask about their hobbies and attempt to identify one we share in common," for example). ("My grandfather is curious about what I've been up to recently, so I'll concentrate on telling him what's new in my life since I last saw him"). Here are some other ways to consider:

Approach #1: Be interested in and curious about other people and make it your aim to discover what makes them intriguing and distinctive.

Approach #2: Discuss the other person's interests.

Approach #3: Determine what subjects you like discussing and then attempt to lead the discussion.

The process of making friends

You've arrived at the chapter's last part, which outlines how to meet friends, develop a social life, and overcome loneliness. Even if you're the kind of person who enjoys spending time alone, you'll feel lonely if your lesser need for social interaction isn't fulfilled. Loneliness may erode your happiness and feeling of self-worth. It's disheartening to spend the seventh Friday night in a row by yourself.

The good news is that learning how to create friends is pretty simple; if you lack an understanding of how to build friendships, you may see some effects right away if you learn and implement the techniques. If you can control your shyness and have a conversation, you should be able to apply the suggestions in this area to enhance your social life.

The fundamentals of building friends:

1. Find potential friends.
2. Invite and plan to do something with those potential friends.
3. Once you've established some new friends, take the relationships to the next level.
4. Repeat the preceding stages until you've created as many friends as possible, whether it's a small group of close friends or a large number.

People who struggle with their social life miss one or more of these stages.

Step 1 - Finding potential friends

The first stage in creating friends is to seek potential friends. That's a prominent place to start, yet it's where some lonely individuals get stuck. They don't expose themselves to enough new prospective pals. This chapter discusses the two primary methods for finding prospects: using your existing connections and meeting new individuals.

Make use of your current contacts

If you've recently moved to a new region and don't know anybody, drawing on your present connections won't work, but you'll frequently find the seeds of social life. You are not required to go out and meet hundreds of people. It is often simpler to convert current connections into full-fledged friends than to find new ones. You could already know a few individuals who might become part of your new social circle.

- Individuals from work or school with whom you get along but have never hung out; acquaintances with whom you're amicable when you run into each other but never see otherwise.
- Friends of individuals you know who you've bonded with when you've met in the past; persons who have shown an interest in becoming your buddy in the past but you never accepted the offer; folks you only meet on occasion but could see more regularly.
- Friends with whom you've lost contact; cousins who live nearby and are your age.

Meet new people

Getting more out of your present relationships might be beneficial, but it isn't always possible. Fortunately, there are many locations where you may meet new individuals. Before we get started, here are some things to bear in mind while looking for new friends.

For instance, you'll probably have to pull yourself out of your routine and prioritize meeting new people. Some lonely individuals slip into a rut where they are comfortable at home when not at work or school.

You may have to try a few different places to meet people before finding one that works for you. Finding new acquaintances is often one of those circumstances when putting in 20% of the work yields 80% of the rewards. You may attend multiple meetups, workshops, or events and find that they are all a flop, but you might easily meet many great people at the next one.

Step 2 – Make a plan for something to do

One early planning stumbling point for some individuals is knowing who they want to hang out with but not knowing where to invite them. It's also very unusual for socially inexperienced individuals to claim that they have no idea what others their age do when they get together. Hanging out with other people is usually about spending time with them.

Don't assume that spending time with somebody is all about planning the perfect event for them to attend. Don't assume there's no purpose in hanging out with them if you can't come up with anything great to do. When you choose to hang out with someone, you are mostly there to enjoy their company. Of course, seeing a band or going on a walk makes your time together more pleasant and memorable, but it's not necessarily required.

Inviting folks to a gathering is frequently more about conducting variants on a few tried-and-true activities than coming up with something unique each time. If you like your friend's company,

112

you may easily spend several weeks hanging out at their place or going to the same rotation of cafés or bars, with just the odd, more exciting event tossed in to change things up.

Create an invitation

After you've decided on an activity, you must ask everyone whether they want to participate.

If someone decides to accept your invitation, it will be because they want to spend time with you and the planned activity interests them, and is accessible. It makes no difference whether you inquired in person, text message, or phone call. Choose the approach that is most convenient for you. On the other hand, group invites are simpler to plan by sending out a single email to which everyone may respond.

Invite folks out in a non-pressuring tone: "It'd be wonderful if you came, but if you don't, that's okay."

Methods for making new friendships

Every friendship is unique, and not every element will relate to every kind in the same way. Some friendships are built on sharing and connecting, while others are built on hobbies, humor, and going out.

- Spend more time with each other.
- Spend one-on-one time with them.
- Maintain contact with them in between hangouts.
- Have a wonderful time while you hang out together.
- Learn more about each other and broaden your conversation subjects. Be a nice friend in all the typical ways.
- Be there for them in their moments of need.
- Have some fun and go on some adventures together.

Have Fulfilling Relationships Without Giving up Who You Are

To have a meaningful relationship, you must devote time and energy to developing the connection and your personal development and self-growth. One cannot exist without the other. The secret formula to having a fulfilling and exciting relationship is to engage in the connection and your own growth. A fulfilling relationship has two parties who invest in their personal growth as much as they do in the partnership's progress.

Small, incremental changes will dramatically revolutionize your relationship. You must take many actions before seeing huge improvements in your relationship. These actions are both beneficial and exciting for the partnership. This enthusiasm motivates you both to make a good life. Not only will your relationship benefit from the minor improvements, but so will you in your personal life.

Live free of expectations.

Don't demand your partner to do anything merely to make you happy.

Wanting your partner to do a certain activity for you to be happy is a toxic way of thinking. How would you feel if your spouse expected you to call as soon as you got home from work? You would probably feel some pressure, and nobody likes feeling forced to do anything. If you didn't feel obligated, you'd be happy to contact your partner after work. Put yourself in your partner's shoes. If you expect your spouse to make you happy constantly, your life will never be truly fulfilled.

A relationship is a link formed by two people who have something to offer each other. You can't expect your spouse to be your

114

only source of happiness. You must take responsibility for your happiness and allow your spouse to contribute. A satisfying relationship occurs when both persons contribute to the enjoyment of the other without any expectations. You are the one who determines whether you are happy or sad. Don't put that choice in the hands of your spouse. Remember that your relationship can only help you be happy.

Concentrate on correcting your flaws.

Instead of pointing out your partner's weaknesses, examine yourself first.

It's our nature to point out the defects of others before examining our own. To have a good relationship, you must recognize the value of concentrating on overcoming your defects rather than pointing out your partner's problems. We all have flaws; it's part of who we are. When you and your partner argue, look inside yourself before focusing on your partner's weaknesses. You will become judgemental and critical if you concentrate too much on your partner's weaknesses. This focus on your partner's weaknesses just erodes the basis of your connection.

Instead of pointing the finger at your spouse the next time you dispute, point the finger at yourself and ask, "What do I need to work on?" It might be the capacity to completely listen to your partner's point of view or the ability to be less obstinate and hardheaded. Whatever the case may be, turn to yourself for the answer rather than your companion. If you continue to concentrate on your partner's weaknesses, you will just be treading water. Make the decision now to begin concentrating on your growth, and this will help not just you but also your relationship.

Keep things cool.

When your spouse does anything that irritates you, don't respond instantly.

Attacking your spouse right away after they have upset you will only make matters worse. Consider the phrase "the quiet before the storm." This is the era of serenity and tranquillity before a period of conflict and sorrow. I know from personal experience how simple it is to lash out at your spouse when they irritate you. Patience and the capacity to deliberately stop oneself from negatively responding are required. It will not be a quick remedy; rather, it will be a long-term behavioral shift. Your actions will either exacerbate or diminish the storm's effect. It's all up to you.

Remember that if you continue to respond to your spouse whenever they upset you negatively, they are more inclined to conceal anything that would upset you. Do you want to build a foundation founded on secrets and lies? I'm certain you don't. Try to take deep breaths and actively prevent yourself from negatively responding. Understand your partner's perspective and communicate in a manner that is successful and promotes constructive discourse. Commit to building a firm foundation of trust, dedication, and patience.

Be interested in your partner.

Whatever problems you face, make it a habit to be interested in your relationship and their needs. I've established this in my own marriage. My spouse and I sit on the sofa every evening after work and ask each other thought-provoking questions. These questions help us both understand each other better. Never let life's stresses take over your relationship. Continue to push back on stress and build the basis of your connection.

Have you ever wondered why young toddlers are so interested in life? They are eager to share what they have learned about the world. A young child's interest and enthusiasm should drive you to do the same with your spouse. Be interested in learning more about your companion. What piques their interest? What brings them joy? What causes them to cry? Questions like these will assist you in creating a vibrant love map of your companion.

Be eager for personal growth.

Maintain a constant flow of ideas about how to grow and develop as an individual and as a pair.

We are all lifetime students. You can learn something new even if you're 87 years old. Every day should be a chance for you to grow, develop, and enhance your life knowledge, and this involves both your development and the growth of your partnership. Read personal development and relationship books to get insights into living a better life.

Did you know that the average commuter in the United States spends 38 hours a year stuck in traffic? Instead of worrying about traffic, listen to an audio program on personal growth or marriage. Listening to an audio program reduces your stress level and increases your knowledge.

The energy of a relationship affects both people. Every day, feed this energy with inspiration. Look for methods to improve yourself and your relationship regularly. Never, ever stop learning because if you stop, you stop developing.

Chapter Nine: Health and Wellbeing

ADHD is defined as difficulty planning and maintaining effort throughout time to attain a good objective in the future under the executive function/motivational deficit hypothesis of ADHD and anxiety. This chapter focuses on the long-term effect of adult ADHD and anxiety on the central aspects of health and well-being management across time.

Although improving health habits cannot be considered therapies for ADHD, unhealthy behaviors may impact ADHD and amplify symptoms of the illness. Therefore, creating healthy habits offers a solid treatment objective and a necessity for an overall wellness approach for treating anxiety and ADHD.

Sleep

People with ADHD who experience anxiety often report difficulties with their sleep's beginning, quantity, and quality. Although most individuals can get through the day after a bad night's sleep, the situation is sometimes more difficult for those with ADHD and anxiety.

The effects on well-being grow more obvious when sleep issues become more regular and persistent. Inadequate sleep is connected with less attention, more distractibility, and more significant problems staying focused in work, lectures, discussions, and awake. It affects numerous other self-regulatory features - the opposite of what people with ADHD and anxiety need.

Furthermore, a disruption of the sleep cycle has a detrimental influence on other biological systems, such as hunger and mood, and is linked to increased cancer risk. The advantages of being a "night person" should be added to the many misconceptions about ADHD, besides "hyperfocus" and "multitasking."

Chronic sleep issues resemble ADHD and anxiety in appearance. In reality, some people with untreated fundamental sleep problems, such as sleep apnea, may wrongly believe they have ADHD or anxiety. In contrast, many people with a history of ADHD and anxiety also have sleep difficulty, with one of these clinical conditions exacerbating the other.

Most people with ADHD and anxiety identify poor sleep as a direct result of ADHD symptoms. The most prevalent challenges are "trouble turning down my thoughts" or "procrastinating on sleep," mainly staying up late to watch television, play computer games, or participate in other online activities despite physical exhaustion. When these conditions continue for a long enough period, the sleep-wake cycle will shift.

Exposure to sunshine helps one remain awake and attentive throughout the day, while the lack of light at night relates to the brain's melatonin production, which aids in sleep. People perform better when they maintain a morning circadian orientation, in which they arise in the morning, are active throughout the day, and sleep at night.

Individuals with ADHD and anxiety have a progressive change to an abnormal evening circadian orientation. This self-identification as a night owl is adopted to rationalize and perpetuate the maladaptive sleep-wake cycle, which affects the body's regulating mechanisms.

As you would expect, getting enough sleep is a critical step in controlling ADHD, and most individuals underestimate the extent to which inadequate sleep impairs performance. Returning to a theme of this guidebook, you likely tell yourself that going to bed at a decent hour is vital. Still, each night, you find yourself remaining online or doing anything else far later than anticipated. Perhaps you've given up on even attempting to go to bed at a reasonable hour. You aim to get more sleep every day, but you don't have a viable strategy.

The first step is to prioritize sleep like a job. That is, rather than describing sleep as being up and busy until you can't keep your eyes open any longer, it becomes a specific activity that you "do" ("I will go to bed at 10 pm").

To determine your bedtime, first determine when you must get up in the morning and then count back by the number of hours you need for a full night's sleep (not the least amount to "get by"), establishing specified sleep and waking periods.

Your daily planner is a tool that helps you to objectively examine your obligations and estimate the time you need to get out of bed every morning to get ready for school, work, or other responsibilities. Even if you do not have an early morning start, such as a scholar whose first class is not until noon or a worker on the second shift, you surely notice that you spend a lot of time in bed yet do not feel rested. We recommend that you set a goal time for beginning your day and arrange your day around that time.

Work backward by eight or nine hours from your actual wake-up time to determine when you should go to bed. There are several exceptions, such as someone who understands that seven hours of sleep is plenty or a working single mother of three children whose obligations do not allow her that much sleep time. You will need to change this number to reflect the reality of your life, but we also urge that you analyze and dispute the notion that "there is no way I can get into bed and fall asleep any sooner." We recommend that you focus on adaptive sleep ideas.

You are an autonomous, free-thinking adult who will make your own choices about how to live your life. However, we urge you to experiment for at least one week – preferably two – to evaluate whether feeling more rested helps you operate better throughout the day. You may discover that what you can achieve during the day—both work/academic and recreational—satisfies you more than what you do late at night rather than sleeping. This experiment requires you to adjust your evening habits and test your belief that you are an unchanging night person.

Consider how you sleep. In truth, sleeping is more of a set of actions you engage in that put your body and brain in a state that permits you to fall asleep. Following the establishment of your goal sleep periods, the next phase in "doing" sleep is breaking the task down into a series of sleep-promoting behavioral tasks that you carry out. These techniques will teach and cue your body and brain to sleep more swiftly and effortlessly over time and with repetition.

A nocturnal regimen is required, just as it is for children. You must also choose a "get into bed" time whenever you choose to begin your sleep cycle. Some individuals know that they fall asleep easily as soon as their head strikes the pillow, and they may not need a ritual other than committing to going to bed. Others need a long time lying in bed before falling asleep because they have difficulty relaxing or quieting their brains.

It is beneficial to have a consistent routine before going to bed to help you wind down your day and prepare for sleep. Start by getting ready for the following day at work or school, packing book bags and meals for the kids, or turning off lights and placing things away. Preparing your coffee maker or putting out the clothing you'll wear to work the following day are fantastic time saves that also help fuel your "sleep script."

We recommend setting aside or disconnecting from computers, smartphones, and devices at least 90 minutes before bed. These devices will prompt justifications for breaking your sleep schedule ("I only need to check a few emails before bed," or "I'll watch one more episode of this show."). There is substantial evidence that the blue light produced by computers, tablets, and smartphone displays fools your brain into thinking it is daytime, interfering with your brain's generation of sleep-promoting melatonin.

In addition to suppressing melatonin, the bright illumination makes it harder to wind down the body's activity and alter body temperature as a component of the sleep onset phase. Delayed Sleep Phase Syndrome affects more than half of individuals with ADHD. On electronic devices, you can employ several applications and other illumination modifications to help wind yourself down if you choose to continue using electronics near bedtime.

Spending time doing something calming will help you fall asleep faster. Many individuals feel that reading fulfills this purpose, while others complain that they get too engrossed in a book. We recommend gathering some go-to sleep reading materials, such as a dull course book, a book with numerous short chapters, or a book you adore but have read so many times that you can simply leave it aside.

You can also use old magazines that you've read multiple times. Some of our patients conduct stretching exercises or light yoga before going to bed. You can also use relaxation techniques before going to bed or lying down.

It is worthwhile to mention a few words about relaxing and managing ADHD and anxiety. We address thoughtful acceptance and the capacity to withstand some pain when confronted with activities, and this guidance also applies to enhancing sleep. You may not feel sleepy after your bedtime routine, but it does not indicate your strategy is ineffective or that you are not exhausted. ADHD impairs your capacity to self-monitor, causing you to be distracted from paying attention to your body and its indications, such as weariness.

The sleep pattern provides a framework for training your brain and body to maintain a better sleep schedule. So, mindful acceptance acknowledges that your body is relaxing even if you are not yet sleeping. Furthermore, resting in bed is more relaxing than doing other things that keep you awake and engaged.

You may practice relaxing techniques while resting in bed. Distracting your mind from day-to-day troubles and controlling your breathing, such as inhaling and exhaling for particular counts, are the basic components of relaxation. That is all that is required.

Having a neutral picture in your mind, such as a color, and gently accepting a troubling notion helps calm your mind. Keeping your breathing pattern slow and regular helps to keep your body calm. To relieve muscular tension, concentrate on relaxing your muscles and allowing your bed to hold you.

These sleep tips – such as having an early cut-off time for caffeine consumption, exercising during the day (but not too close to bedtime), and not watching the clock if you wake up during the night – are all things you can do to enhance your sleep and reboot your circadian schedule. If you take a stimulant medication for ADHD or anxiety, you should talk to your doctor about the time of your final dosage and how it can influence your sleep.

You must:

1. Make sleep a top priority.
2. Establish the time you must be up in the morning.
3. Work backward from the number of hours of sleep you need to determine when you should go to bed. Write down this sleep time in your daily planner.

4. Create a sleep pattern that encourages you to enter "sleep mode." This pattern might involve arranging your clothing and other belongings for the following day, putting away devices 90 minutes before bed, reading or indulging in other soothing activities, etc.

5. Follow conventional sleep hygiene rules throughout the day, such as no coffee after a certain time, limiting alcohol usage, sleeping exclusively in your bed, avoiding activity too late in the day, keeping the bedroom at a suitable temperature, and limiting daytime naps, etc.

6. Be aware of sleep-related cognitive mistakes. Even if you get a bad night's sleep, you will have enough energy the following day to perform effectively, even if you are not at your best.

7. If you wake up at night, avoid looking at the time.

8. If you have trouble falling back asleep, get out of bed for ten minutes and read or sit quietly before returning to bed.

Exercise

It will be no surprise that exercise has several health advantages, including enhanced sleep. Exercise has been linked to specific advantages for individuals with ADHD and anxiety, such as time-limited increases in concentration and mood. Exercise can reverse – and ideally avoid – certain concerning health patterns observed in research that follows children with ADHD as they enter adulthood.

Aside from continuing ADHD symptoms into adulthood, these people have risk factors for coronary heart disease due to their lifestyle choices. Although these trends are not conclusive, individuals with ADHD are more likely to have sedentary lifestyles, have poor eating habits, and participate in harmful activities such as nicotine use. Correspondingly, you should find a strategy to maintain a healthy level of exercise.

Let us distinguish between health and fitness. It is possible to be healthy without being physically fit. The purpose of exercise does not have to improve one's physical fitness or athletic ability, while these are good goals that inspire some individuals. Rather, we hope you outline a realistic health habit in particular words, concentrate on the initial steps to get started, and then make appointments with yourself to carry out this plan (with a start time and an end time). Presumably, you will be able to build and maintain this fitness routine over time.

Simple, quick, and inexpensive is a technique to find plans that you are more likely to start and maintain. Walking is a simple habit that most individuals can adopt. There are numerous ways to begin a walking plan without significantly altering your current routine. These include taking the stairs at work, walking to work, walking during breakfast or other breaks, or taking your dog for a long walk when you get home from work.

Committing to someone else, like walking your dog or organizing walks with a colleague or spouse, encourages follow-through and strengthens connections. Signing up for a yoga class or joining a softball team, for example, holds you responsible for others and enhances the probability that you will stick to your plan. You may prefer alternative types of exercise, such as biking or going to the gym three days a week. The goal is to discover an activity or a menu of activities that you can stick with.

"I don't have time" is a common justification for not beginning an exercise routine. Rather than assuming this, study your daily planner and ask yourself, "When do I have time to squeeze in some exercise?" Again, defining the sort of activity in mind is beneficial. Even if you can't afford the time or money to attend the gym, you can find ways to get some extra walking in throughout the day, even if it means taking the stairs instead of the elevator at work or parking at the far end of the parking lot at work or a shop.

Of course, exercising is one of those jobs that are especially prone to procrastination and a slew of negative ideas like "I'm too tired," "I'm not in the game to work out," and "I'll do it tomorrow." We often use exercise as an example to illustrate typical procrastination circumstances and cognitions (independent of ADHD status).

Identifying and challenging these procrastinating ideas is critical: "I'm exhausted after work, but I know that I'll feel better and more invigorated once I get started," she says. "No one is ever in the mood to work out." "Let me concentrate on turning off the TV, getting up, and changing into my workout clothes," and "I'm exaggerating the drawbacks of exercise while discounting the rewards." "I'll exercise for at least 15 minutes, and if that's all I can do today, I'll call it a day." Remembering and factoring in the great sensations you receive throughout the exercise and the joy of finishing it is beneficial.

People frequently ask us how long it takes for a habit to form. We cannot offer a clear answer, but we have discovered that two weeks—two work weeks and two weekends—is a reasonable baseline. We advise you to test a healthy activity, such as a daily walk, to see whether it may become more regular and need less effort to accomplish.

Healthy Eating

Maintaining healthy eating habits is a fantastic strategy to enhance general health and provide the groundwork for improved ADHD and anxiety management. Food choices, paying close attention to when and how much you eat, and coping with impulsivity are aspects of good eating pertinent to ADHD and anxiety. Individuals on stimulant drugs for ADHD or anxiety may experience appetite suppression, a frequent adverse effect of this type of medication.

Reduced appetite in children or teenagers using ADHD meds needs close monitoring to ensure they obtain adequate calories and nutrients. Young people, especially those in college, must be cautious of their diets and food consumption. Even if there is no health or nutrition problem, poor self-monitoring, planning, and impulsivity may lead to an overreliance on unhealthy convenience meals. Adults with ADHD and anxiety may also underestimate the impact of increased hunger and blood sugar drops on mood, impulsive control, and focus.

It is beneficial to ensure that you have something to eat at each of the three conventional meal times, even if it is a modest quantity. Similarly, keeping nutritious snacks nearby, such as crackers or granola bars, can supply you with enough nutrition and energy to keep you going until you can have a real meal or at least a more substantial snack.

Staying hydrated is another key issue since inadequate self-monitoring may put you at risk for dehydration, making you feel ill even in moderate cases. Because the dry mouth is a typical side effect of many drugs, water provides a simple, healthful, zero-calorie alternative.

When it comes to healthy eating, stimulus management is key. Making educated decisions about the foods you have on hand is a sort of environmental engineering. If you don't have any ice cream in your freezer, you don't have to decide whether to eat that late-night bowl of ice cream. These procedures need planning to locate healthy alternatives (like crunchy fruit instead of crunchy potato chips). Include these appropriate health behavior activities in your overall coping strategy.

We don't want you to have an all-or-nothing attitude toward eating or believe that individuals with ADHD and anxiety can't have certain guilty pleasures. However, you must be cautious not to exploit

Ben Franklin's motto, "moderation in all things—including moderation," to justify reckless action. You can adjust your eating habits despite allegations that you are a "junk food addict," just as you can create sleep patterns after becoming a night person.

We recommend that you begin the change process by concentrating on a single implementation goal, enhancing one healthy habit and lowering one problematic behavior. For example, for one week, purchase apples (or a variety of fruits) as your healthy snack instead of potato chips (or other bad snack food). Another option is to make a healthy substitution within a snack meal, such as unbuttered microwave popcorn instead of the mega-ultra theatre-artery-clogging-style-butter type.

Similarly to overcoming procrastination to begin work, you will likely discover that you have increased your eating pleasure in a healthy alternative after choosing a healthy option. The goal is not to exclude everything but the most nutritious items from your diet but instead to make educated eating choices, modify your eating habits in a better direction, and reduce the negative impacts of impulsivity on your well-being.

Harmful Habits and How to Change Them

ADHD and anxiety are linked to an increased risk of drug use disorders, notably alcohol, marijuana, or nicotine use. Caffeine may also be used excessively, with many young people utilizing highly caffeinated energy drinks to self-medicate symptoms and to remain up to combat the consequences of poor sleep patterns.

Several paths lead to the formation of these undesirable behaviors. Your family of origin may have exposed you to these behaviors, indicating a hereditary predisposition for drug abuse. Peer pressure may magnify impulsivity, leading to teenage drug use and continuing as self-medicine for the undiagnosed ADHD. Whatever the cause, these habits cause issues in your life and make managing ADHD much more difficult.

In a full-fledged drug or alcohol addiction, the first step is to seek treatment for the addiction via a detoxification program. It is believed that 25% of people in treatment programs have a background of ADHD. Even though ADHD is the apparent cause that puts you at risk for these issues, you need to be clean and sober before treating the ADHD symptoms with drugs, psychosocial therapy, or other methods. A history of addiction and the possibility of associated mood or anxiety disorders complicates your clinical position and treatment demands, including monitoring your risk of relapse.

Most readers' drug use, if it occurs at all, will not be of the frequency or volume that necessitates inpatient recovery or even comes close to being termed an addiction. However, you may notice certain troublesome behaviors that interfere with your ability to control ADHD and serve as distractions or escape routes. Thus, you may use marijuana or alcohol to cope with stress or racing thoughts when trying to sleep. Still, these behaviors may also keep you trapped in a cycle of procrastination, denial, and under-function. Likewise, excessive dependence on nicotine or caffeine may improve your capacity to concentrate on a task in the short term, but it may have health consequences that exceed the advantages.

Recognizing these harmful practices as contributing to your coping issues is the first step in dealing with your ADHD more directly. Once in therapy, these behaviors are often targeted for correction. Medications for ADHD that lower fundamental symptoms should help you better handle activities. You won't need to use drugs to escape the tension and other emotions.

You must:

1. Get enough sleep.
2. Prioritize a decent amount of activity/exercise in your daily schedule.
3. Concentrate on developing at least one good eating behavior and eliminating one harmful eating habit.
4. Plan and track your health activities using your daily planner.
5. Be proactive in obtaining care for changes in symptoms caused by menstrual cycles, pregnancy, early menopause, or menopause in women.
6. Engage in safe sex, including birth control devices that protect against sexually transmitted diseases.
7. Monitor and make efforts (including seeking therapy) to eliminate harmful habits, such as nicotine and excessive caffeine use.

Final Thoughts

We've discussed the definition, causes, and treatments for social anxiety. This book has provided simple yet solid and practical ways for dealing with social anxiety and ADHD, allowing you to make changes in your life that will bring you peace and pleasure. You've also learned a little bit about my own life and how I'm now using my experiences to assist others.

You now understand what social anxiety is and how powerful it can be in a person's life. You should also understand the notion that happy thoughts attract favorable outcomes, while negative mental pictures just serve to bring more negativity into your life. You've also discovered that you can construct your own life and that your ideas shape the life you live.

You must use all of the information and practices you have read in this book for it to be effective. You must utilize all of them, even if they are not in the sequence we have listed in this book.

You are now aware of the need to know and have decided to conquer social anxiety by writing down your goals for your life. The next step would be to request what you want. It is critical to believe in what you desire and have decided on, and you should not allow any doubts to seep in afterward.

Always think about what you want and think positively. Any negative thinking will erode the gains you've accomplished. Last but not least, you now understand the power of thankfulness. Always express gratitude for everything in your life. More importantly, keep in mind that you must strive and act toward your intended objectives for the transition to be effective. No miracles exist.

Begin immediately with small actions that will enable you to apply the tactics to your advantage properly. Undoubtedly, conquering social anxiety is proven to alter lives; it is up to you to choose an area of your life or what you desire and request the universe to begin the process of transformation. Make more inquiries and do other research to broaden your understanding of social anxiety and the strategies presented here.

You must have a clear mind to benefit from this book. You must cultivate habits that will assist you in achieving your aim for mental clarity, leaving you healthier, happier, and more successful. You will obtain success, pleasure, personal satisfaction, and excellent health by thinking clearly.

When you can't think clearly, you often make bad judgments. Anxiety develops due to being continually doubtful or concerned, and the resulting stress leads to ill health. Indeed, clear thinking is essential for personal happiness and wellness.

You must discover how to enhance your health for improved mental clarity by cultivating your existing abilities and making changes in your life that obscure your judgment. Clear thinking has been characterized as the capacity to think clearly and intelligently without being confused. It is being rational. Clear thinking, in my opinion, is having the presence of mind to successfully regulate your ideas, examine your thoughts, and ultimately make solid judgments.

To be a clear thinker, you must be able to process thoughts logically and in depth via independent and reflective thinking. It is more than just information acquisition since it does not only rely on memory. For increased knowledge and intelligent judgments, you must be capable of anticipating the implications of what you know.

Furthermore, clear thinking encompasses much more than just thinking; it comprises mental nurture, wellness, and the structuring of our life. Our ideas or thoughts ultimately decide who we become. Every day, you make various choices with far-reaching repercussions, all of which stem from the same source—your mind. Mental clarity and wellness are essential for making sound judgments. Clear thinking necessitates clear thinking. When your mind is congested, you are on edge and preoccupied, and you do very little.

A lot is going on in someone's head. As a result, you do not need to keep everything in your head. Get a tool to help you keep track of everything. This tool should function as a storage device for any information you do not want to forget. For instance, if you have an appointment or a future project, write it down or note it in your calendar. You might also maintain a more thorough diary. A notebook will allow you to get rid of everything that keeps you from getting things done, such as relationship issues, providing you peace of mind.

Let go of memories of errors made, individuals we have harmed, previous disappointments, and wasted chances. Most individuals cling to these memories and refuse to let them go. Memories that bring you down clog your mind and life, preventing you from thinking clearly.

When you decide to tackle a job, begin with the essential one and work your way down the list until the last one is completed. Take on no more than one job at a time, then set aside a certain amount of time to arrange everything. During that time, keep your thoughts clean and set aside everything that can distract you from work at hand.

Too much knowledge might clog your mind. This information that you take in daily from periodicals, newspapers, television, social media sites and the internet must be regulated. You may restrict the quantity of information you consume by determining how much time you devote to social media and other sources. Unsubscribe from online magazines and blogs that are of no use to you. Consider ideas from people you respect, and ultimately, disregard extraneous information.

Create a schedule for every part of your life and everything you do. This schedule will assist in lessening the amount of stress your brain has to deal with. Plan for the minor details ahead of time. Complete several tasks daily. You cannot, however, do everything. Make a list of the essential items and deal with them. It gives your mind time and space to think clearly.

Mental clutter obstructs our inner thoughts and stands in the way of clear thinking and focusing on what is essential. Begin by emptying your thoughts of useless items that take up mental space but bring no value or boost clear thinking.

Personal transformation must begin at the subconscious level; else, it will never occur. Improving our review is the key to changing our life and attaining what we want. Working on the subconscious to alter your thinking is as easy as imagining what you desire and concentrating on it for some time.

Working on the subconscious will almost certainly unlock the hidden power of your subconscious mind and help you acquire what you desire when you allow yourself. You're intended to attract things rather than chase them down, and the subconscious mind is the key to making that happen.

References

Cuncic, A. (2021, February 19). Understanding the causes of social anxiety disorder. Verywell Mind. Retrieved May 18, 2022, from https://www.verywellmind.com/social-anxiety-disorder-causes-3024749

Hallowell, E. M., & Ratey, J. J. (2022). Adhd 2.0: New science and essential strategies for thriving with distraction--from childhood through adulthood. Ballantine Books.

Koyuncu, A., Ertekin, E., Yüksel, Ç., Aslantaş Ertekin, B., Çelebi, F., Binbay, Z., & Tükel, R. (2015). Predominantly inattentive type of ADHD is associated with social anxiety disorder. Journal of attention disorders, 19(10), 856-864.

Rodebaugh, T. L., Holaway, R. M., & Heimberg, R. G. (2004). The treatment of social anxiety disorder. Clinical Psychology Review, 24(7), 883-908.

Stein, M. B., & Stein, D. J. (2008). Social anxiety disorder. The Lancet, 371(9618), 1115-1125.

Weiss, G., & Hechtman, L. T. (1993). Hyperactive children grown up: ADHD in children, adolescents, and adults. Guilford Press.

Çelebi, F., & Ünal, D. (2021). Self esteem and clinical features in a clinical sample of children with ADHD and social anxiety disorder. Nordic Journal of Psychiatry, 75(4), 286-291.

ADHD 2.0

EFFECT ON MARRIAGE

Target 7 Days

Turn Anger into Love

Overcome Anxiety in Relationship | Couple Conflicts | Insecurity in Love

Improve Communication Skills | Empath & Psychic Abilities.

Margaret Hampton

Introduction

Are you in a marriage that sometimes feels more like a relationship between a parent and a child? Do you feel like one of you is taking on a larger burden of care and it's straining your partnership? Is one or both of you forgetful or disorganized to the point of dysfunction? Does your house always feel like a reflection of the mess that is your life?

If all this feels almost painfully familiar, you may be in an ADHD-affected relationship. ADHD affects somewhere between 4 and 6 percent of adults and it's been found that ADHD-affected marriages end in divorce at nearly twice the rate of non-affected marriages. That doesn't mean there's no hope for you and your partner, though. It can seem intimidating to tackle a problem that feels so large and leaves you both feeling like everything is out of control. This book is designed to help you understand more about the disorder and how it affects relationships. We're going to take you through seven days of work to get your marriage back on track, help eliminate the insecurities and anxieties that stem from the disorder, and build your love and empathy for each other back to where it was when you first fell in love.

We'll start by learning more about what ADHD is and isn't, and what traits of ADHD are affecting your marriage. This book aims to help both the affected and non-affected spouses. You can work together or you can apply the techniques and tips you've learned on your own.

Day One will look at turning your frustration around. It could feel overwhelming being constantly upset at the things that your spouse does. You blame them or blame yourself for the issues in your relationship, but you can learn to turn those negative feelings back into feelings of love and compassion.

Day Two will help you overcome the anxieties that crop up in relationships with ADHD. Sometimes it can seem like the disorder turns our partner into the Incredible Hulk. They can be quick to anger or quick to respond with strong emotion, which can leave you feeling confused and upset. Other times feel like they're ignoring you to focus on something that seems insignificant to you. Are they spending hours and hours on their hobbies or interests? You'll learn how to understand them better and how to fix things when you feel the distance growing.

Day Three will look at how the disorder can affect people's ability to form secure attachments and how they may struggle with the social skills necessary for a successful relationship. You'll learn how to help your affected spouse with their relationship skills and better understand each other's nonverbal cues. We will also include tips for couples who struggle with interpersonal relationships outside the home and how to navigate those situations as a couple.

Day Four will have you learning more about the conflict that arises in relationships with an affected partner and how to manage conflict within the relationship. Sometimes the disorder can affect how you deal with conflict in the relationship. You'll learn how to become more comfortable with conflict when necessary and become a better listener and a better problem solver.

Day Five will be all about improving your communication skills. Sometimes within an ADHD-affected marriage, it can be difficult for the non-affected spouse to get their point across to the ADHD-affected spouse. We'll look at some solutions to common communication issues and when to seek outside help for the relationship.

Day Six will focus on how to eliminate the insecurities in your relationships. In addition, we will delve into ways to improve the affected spouse's self-esteem and build confidence in the relationship, and how to communicate constructive feedback effectively.

Day Seven will be all about fostering empathy and love for each other. You'll learn how to become more empathetic, and ways to fall in love all over again after the issues around the disorder have strained your relationship. You'll also learn about your affected partner's qualities that can actually make your marriage better and how to nurture those qualities in your spouse.

When learning about how the disorder affects your marriage, the first step is to understand more about ADHD and what it is. Attention Deficit/Hyperactive Disorder is a neurological disorder that has no defined cause as of yet. It's thought to be caused by a combination of factors such as environment, genetics, and fetal development. It's most often thought of as a disorder that affects young boys, but there are still a significant number of girls and women affected by ADHD. Unfortunately, for various reasons, the disorder goes underdiagnosed in women to this day.

It is a spectrum disorder, and there are three primary types: Hyperactive-Impulsive, Inattentive, and Combination. Boys are more likely to be diagnosed with Hyperactive-Impulsive while girls are more likely to be diagnosed with Inattentive type ADHD. Both genders can experience any of the three types, though.

Some of the symptoms include:

- Impulsive behaviors
- Poor time management skills
- Issues focusing on a task
- Trouble with multitasking
- Disorganization and problems prioritizing

- Frequent moods swings
- Low tolerance for external stimuli
- Low tolerance for frustration
- Restlessness or excessive energy
- Inability to sit still
- Difficulty coping with stress
- Emotional dysregulation
- Short attention span
- Appearing forgetful or frequently losing things
- Being easily distracted
- Poor organization

It can feel frustrating to deal with a spouse who seems to have the attention span of a goldfish. You feel like you're constantly repeating information you think they should remember. You might be experiencing frustration with their impulsive behaviors or even get upset when their impulses lead them to make decisions such as financing a new car when there's a baby on the way. It can feel like their inability to stay organized means you have to carry the load of the household duties, lest nothing gets done.

These are all common symptoms of the disorder. They can be managed with things like medication, therapy, and exercise. Even if they are not properly managed, there are ways that you, as the non-affected spouse, can help your affected spouse cope with the difficulties that the disorder brings. The two of you can work together to create a better, more fulfilling relationship!

We have seven days to turn things around. So let's start with day one.

Day One: Turn Frustration Into Love

Exercise: Sit together in a neutral space, such as the living room or on the porch. Avoid doing this in intimate spaces like the bedroom or personal spaces like your home office. Light a candle. Each of you will then take turns making "I feel" statements to each other about your current frustrations, such as "I feel frustrated that I'm doing most of the cooking lately and it's getting tiring for me." Acknowledge each other's feelings. Don't agree or disagree; just acknowledge how your partner feels at that moment.

After letting out your feelings, blow out the candle. The candle will symbolize releasing your frustrations and letting go of anger. You can now talk through your "I feel" statements if you want, but during the exercise, the point is to give each other space to listen and feel heard.

The disorder comes with a host of symptoms that, believe it or not, can directly affect your ability to navigate relationships healthily. In addition, symptoms can cause misunderstandings, frustration, and resentment on the part of either partner. These symptoms can be difficult to deal with in everyday life but can be damaging in a relationship.

When you're a person with ADHD, it might feel like your partner is hypercritical or constantly nagging you about your household chores. You don't feel respected or treated as an equal; you even start to feel as though you're being treated like a child. It can feel like your significant other wants to micromanage you, and you start to wonder if the relationship is worth the struggles. You feel frustrated that nothing you do seems to be right. No matter what, you feel like you're constantly making mistakes or doing things the wrong way.

Being constantly berated by your spouse might bring up bad childhood memories–memories of being bullied or looked down on for being different. Maybe you went into this marriage thinking you finally met someone who understands you and accepts you, but now you're questioning if that's still true. People with this disorder are often more sensitive to criticism, especially if they feel like they've been criticized their entire lives for not being "normal" enough. This is definitely something that can lead to insecurities building up over time. You wonder if your spouse thinks you're good enough, and it might wear on your self-esteem.

For the non-affected spouse, you feel ignored when you make requests. You get lonely when your spouse gets hyper-fixated on a project or frustrated at the amount of time they spend on their hobby, leading to resentment from feeling neglected and like you're carrying more of the emotional labor. You might also be getting upset when you feel like you're the only reliable partner in the relationship. It can get exhausting wondering if they will follow through on their promises. It can start to feel like they just don't care.

It could be extremely tough if you went into the marriage with expectations that your partner would get better. No one should go into a marriage expecting their partner to change, but it happens. You might have believed that once the affected spouse "settled down," they would take adult responsibilities more seriously, especially when children become involved in the equation.

These frustrations can be understandable. Dealing with them is probably exhausting for both partners. It's easy to blame the affected spouse. Still, with a deeper understanding of how the disorder works and the common problems that can arise in a relationship with someone affected by the disorder, you will be able to eliminate those

145

frustrations. Let's go over the symptoms of ADHD again, specifically the ones that most affect relationships:

- **Trouble paying attention**: Having this disorder might mean you zone out during conversations, miss important details, or agree to something you later forget about. You feel like you're trying to pay attention but you can easily become distracted in a busy environment. You aren't trying to ignore your partner or forget what they said, but it might feel that way to them. You feel as though you have tried to explain this but it can be frustrating to someone who is neurotypical because they may not fully understand how difficult it can be.

- **Forgetfulness**: It can feel like even when your partner *is* paying attention, they end up forgetting what was discussed anyway. It might seem like the only important things to *them* are those they remember, but that's not true. ADHD brains can store long-term memories without issue but struggle with retaining short-term memories. That's why they might be able to recite pi to the one-hundredth digit but can't seem to remember to pick up cat litter on the way home from work.

- **Emotional outbursts**; People with ADHD have a harder time with emotional regulation. Their brains can't properly process emotional responses and strong emotions can overwhelm them until they're bursting. For people with this disorder, it can feel like your body gets hot when you're angry or upset, and for your partner, it may feel like they are walking on eggshells to keep from upsetting you.

- **Poor organizational skills**: Having the disorder is like a constant whirlwind in your head. It can be hard to keep track of your own thoughts, let alone all the tasks necessary to keep a household going. It may feel like the affected spouse is just lazy or disorganized, but in reality, there's a lot more going on. It can certainly be frustrating though, to feel like the majority of household tasks fall to you. The ADHD-affected partner may feel frustrated and guilty at the way their partner feels and lash out as a defense.
- **Impulsivity**: ADHD-related impulsivity can be a struggle. Sometimes you have no brain-to-mouth filter. You end up thoughtlessly blurting out something hurtful without realizing it. Your brain craves the rush of dopamine that comes from instant gratification and wants you to spend recklessly or you crave addictive behaviors. This can affect your relationship with your partner in many ways, from financial stress to your spouse feeling that you put your addictions above your family.

The first step to overcoming some of the frustrations that come from dealing with this disorder, either as the affected partner or the neurotypical partner, is to understand how each of you is feeling when dealing with these issues. Are you stressed carrying the majority of the household duties? Do you feel like you're juggling a dozen plates in the air at all times and if you let one plate drop, the entire thing will come crashing down? Do you feel like you can't rely on your affected partner and they are adding to your stress?

You probably try to give your partner advice. You offer solutions. You send them reminders. Nothing seems to work. You feel like they are ignoring you on purpose. When you need encouragement or a positive compliment, you feel like that seems always to be the

147

moment your partner blurts out something rude or off-putting. You feel like they go out of their way to hit you where it hurts during your arguments. It can feel like they are going out of their way to upset you.

Carrying the emotional load can be hard. You might be at your wit's end, feeling as if nothing you do is getting through to your partner, as if nothing will ever change. That can be an exhausting experience. As you struggle with the issues caused by the disorder, it can feel like your ability to desire and love your partner is waning. It might feel like you don't know how to connect emotionally anymore. When your affected partner chooses to engage for hours on a hyper fixation or spends weeks or months of their free time focused on a project instead of connecting with you, you can start to question their loyalty and devotion. No matter how much you beg, plead, threaten, cajole, discuss or yell, nothing changes. You even start to feel like you're on the verge of a breakdown.

It can be hard on the non-affected spouse, for sure. However, it can often be just as difficult for the affected partner. They have their own emotional turmoil. It can feel like you are the only one feeling frustrated, but the problems are a two-way street.

ADHD can be a stressful disorder. You're sensitive to many kinds of stimuli whether that be noises, textures, foods, or smells. It can be overwhelming trying to process throughout the day. Managing daily life can also be much more work than others realize. People with this disorder often experience the world uniquely, which others may not understand. You feel like you're almost speaking a different language to your partner, trying to explain how things work for you. It can feel like you'll never live up to others' expectations. You feel like you're constantly making mistakes or failing at things you set out to do. You could be overcompensating with humor or lashing out in anger to hide your true feelings. When bombarded by criticisms from your partner, your boss, family, and friends, you can start to feel like

148

people don't care about you, just the person they want you to be. You feel like your failure to live up to expectations pushes your partner away. You can start to feel like they don't want you around and rebuff your attempts at connection. The more times you fail to meet expectations, the more fear you have of the consequences. You become too afraid even to try anymore. One of the strongest desires for people with ADHD is to be accepted. You might be longing for your partner to love you for who you are despite your imperfections.

There are many ways symptoms can affect your relationships, but these are the most common areas likely to give you trouble and cause a significant strain. The frustrations may have built up to the point where you and your partner feel a divide that can't be bridged. It doesn't have to stay like that, however. Medication and therapy are good ways to help. There are also ways to cross that divide with techniques that you can use together, right at home. Here are a few techniques to help you and your partner avoid or overcome some of the problems that arise with ADHD:

For the non-affected partner

When you're getting stressed out by your spouse's actions, you're more likely to lash out at them. All the nagging and verbal confrontations in the world haven't helped so far and will continue to make your spouse feel more defensive than helped. Time to learn to let go and know you can only control yourself. Use positive reinforcement with them. It might feel unnecessary or condescending but saying something like, "Hey, thanks for taking the trash out today! I meant to ask, but you beat me to it!" goes a long way towards positively reinforcing the behavior you want to see. Acknowledge their efforts and achievements. Letting them know you're proud of them for sticking with a new routine or habit can also help them in the long run.

On the other hand, don't go so far as to act like their parent. It can feel like nagging your partner is what works, but treating them as a child or being condescending can damage your relationship and destroy their self-esteem. Communicate the issue and then let them deal with the consequences if they are unable or unwilling to follow through. Don't take over their duties either. You'll only grow in your resentment the more you take on. Try to focus on their intentions instead of their shortcomings. It may feel like they're ignoring you when they lose concentration but remember, it's not about you; it's their brain. You feel as though your partner finds you uninteresting, but they likely don't mean to make you feel unloved.

For the affected partner

Start by acknowledging what's happening. Your partner might not be communicating in a way that you like, but the fact is, your issues *are* interfering in your relationship. You need to acknowledge that the problem isn't solely on your partner to fix you and your issues, that it's on you as well. You are a team, and you can't expect your partner to act as your manager. If you know that a conversation is turning into an argument or that a situation provokes strong emotions in you, have an agreed-upon code word that you two use when things are getting out of your control. Use the code word to signal to your partner that you two need to take a break from the conversation or situation until you can calm down and regroup. Pick something that wouldn't come up in everyday conversation, such as "Kumquat" or "Ollivander."

When your spouse feels cared for, even with small gestures, that can go a long way towards making them feel more valued. When they go out of their way to take care of an issue you've been struggling with, don't get upset! Show them gratitude and understand that they're only trying to help. You know you have ADHD. Are you utilizing all the help and resources to manage your condition? Are you exploring treatment options and looking up ways to help yourself in your weak spots? If you don't have a toolbox of tools to use, you're not being fair to your partner. Once you start learning to manage the symptoms that make life more difficult for you and your partner, life will become smoother.

The two of you should work together to pick ways to mitigate stress. Do things like having a no-chores day. Yes, it's important to keep up with the housework, but it can sometimes feel like a lot of your problems revolve around the division of labor or who is and isn't doing their fair share. Pick one day a week that you both agree on that remains a chore-free day. It might feel stressful at first to let go, but you should both focus on quality time or enjoy free time to do things you might not normally get to do. Whether that's simply binge-watching a show together or spending time on your hobbies in the same room, do something that you enjoy and doesn't revolve around responsibility.

Sometimes when the two of you are having a conflict or disagreement and tensions are high, you can feel like you're simply angry or frustrated. Take a step back to identify the heart of the emotion. There's a saying that there are only two emotions: love and fear. This is simplistic, but, when it comes down to it, maybe as the non-affected partner, you fear that your partner will never step up and you'll be alone in the relationship. Perhaps as the affected partner, you fear your partner getting fed up and leaving you. You're both coming from the same place–the fear of being alone. Real love isn't a feeling so much as it's an action. It can be difficult to choose your partner day in and day out, especially when they're driving you to frustration, but you picked that person for a reason. Take a few minutes out of your day, both of you, to sit and list five things you like about your partner. You don't have to say them out loud to each other (though that can be helpful), but it will help you remember that there are qualities you love about them.

Of course, sometimes, it can get to the point where it feels like nothing is changing. Maybe you are in a rut, and an outside opinion can help. There are many options–everything from seeing your spiritual advisor if you belong to a religious group to going to a licensed family counselor. If cost is an issue, there are many free or sliding-scale options out there. You both need to go into the session with open minds and let go of the idea that the blame rests solely on one person. When trying to turn the relationship around and improve your conflict-resolution skills, it can help to step back and put yourself in your partner's shoes. Think about the way your partner might feel in reaction to your statements. Think through how they might be feeling about the situation. You can gain a lot of clarity if you take that time to recognize and acknowledge their perspective.

You and your partner might be spending a lot of time misinterpreting each other's actions and intentions. When you're disagreeing, you could be assigned your interpretation to what you're hearing without giving your partner the benefit of the doubt. For example, when the non-ADHD affected partner says, "When you spend all day working on the car, I feel like I have to take care of the kids by myself," this may come across as accusations of being lazy to the affected partner. Instead, practice active listening. When your partner makes a statement, repeat your understanding of their words. This will allow them to clarify their intent and meaning.

When dealing with this disorder, there's one really great way to approach any problem that arises. For those affected, it may be difficult to do things the "normal" or "usual" way, and you need to adapt and change your approach, finding what works. If it feels stupid, but it works, it's not stupid. For the non-affected partner, you're going to have to get past the idea that your partner "should" do things a certain way, or you're going to drive a wedge trying to make the affected spouse live up to your expectations.

Don't forget to lean into the unconventional and find humor in dealing with the situation. Sometimes, you have to laugh at just how absurd life with a chronic condition can be. Learning to laugh at the silly miscommunications and the wild misunderstandings can help you both relieve some of the tension and even bring you closer together. When you get the urge to impulsively say something negative, use an imaginary key or mime zipping your mouth up so you don't blurt out something hurtful. When tensions are high or stress is piling up, take time out of your schedules to work out. Take a walk, do yoga, or have a mini dance party. Get up and moving as exercise gives you endorphins that can help combat stress and fatigue. It also has a positive effect on ADHD, helping to calm the brain and improve focus.

If communicating face-to-face is difficult or causes strong emotional reactions, write down the things you want to say to each other via email. It gives you the space to sort out your feelings and can be a good way to express the things you have a hard time saying. Alternatively, send each other kind and loving emails once a day or once a week to remind each other how much you care. It doesn't need to be long, but it should be thoughtful. Also, getting educated on ADHD and its symptoms and difficulties means understanding how it's affecting your relationship. It's good for both partners–the affected partner might learn new techniques that help manage their symptoms and make life easier, and the non-affected spouse might be able to take the challenges less seriously. Check in once a week with each other to have the opportunity to discuss any issues and celebrate the progress you two have made. Use it as an opportunity to grow as a couple. Lastly, sometimes you have to give up on the idea that it should always fall to the two of you to take care of everything. Instead, outsource help or delegate tasks. For example, get groceries delivered, assign your children age-appropriate chores and set up automatic drafts for bills. These will eliminate a lot of the worries and stresses that you face.

It will take work to move from daily frustrations back to love and empathy. There are going to be missteps along the way. You may feel like it's two steps forward and one step back some days. It's okay to be frustrated. It's okay to feel your feelings. It's not about achieving perfect harmony, total balance, and complete serenity. It's about finding ways to work with the tools you have to create the lives you want for yourselves. When you use your tools, you're less likely to feel as though you can't do it–you know you're empowered enough to get it done. You don't have to be perfect; you just have to learn how to embrace your imperfections. With ADHD, you have hyperfocus– this can help you in so many ways.

The best way to start is to create an action plan. Come up with a way that the two of you will work together; using the tips above to make a change for the better. When you have a plan in place, you have something to fall back on when things repeatedly start to slip out of control. For example, you struggle with setting up organizational systems. Your partner can step in here and offer assistance with coming up with ideas that work for both of you. Remember, if it's stupid, but it works, it's not stupid.

Start by analyzing the areas in which you two have the most conflict. Do you struggle with your partner remembering to do the things that you ask? Is your partner chronically late? Does the division of labor feel unfair? Next, come up with practical, actionable solutions. For things like forgotten requests, stick a post-it note inside your partner's lunchbox, text them a reminder before they leave work, or write them on a dry erase board by the door. For chronic lateness, set up calendar reminders that you can share across your phones, set timers for yourself if you know you underestimate how much time you have, and make sure you work backward on timing–add in everything from getting ready to walking out the door to finding parking.

If chores are going undone, develop a routine. Having a daily routine in place will help you both to remember what needs to get done that day. Start with the morning and work your way through to the evening, developing a list of what you do all day. For instance, you usually wake up at eight, then eat breakfast, brush your teeth, get dressed, and feed the dog. Writing it down will help you remember so you don't have to mentally remember it. It may seem silly, but you'll associate each step with the next one by writing all the steps down. You'll be less likely to forget to brush your teeth if you know you do it after eating breakfast. You'll remember to feed the dog because that comes directly after brushing your teeth.

Additionally, set up a system for controlling the clutter in the house. Less clutter means less anxiety which means less avoidance of tasks. Get baskets for the stairs or the living room where you put all the stuff that doesn't go there. Drop it in the basket, and when it's full, clear it out by putting things away. Do the dishes immediately after dinner instead of waiting so you aren't as likely to put it off. After eating breakfast, put the dishes away in the drainer first so they don't sit there all day. Come up with ways that work with your ADHD, and you'll be less likely to be overwhelmed by the amount of mess or clutter around you.

When it comes to remembering questions, repeat what your partner said and what you agreed to do. That ensures that you both know you were listening and are more likely to remember the task the way it was intended. Write it down on a post-it, in your planner or as a note on your phone so that you don't forget either. Set a reminder using an app on your phone to go off when it's time to do the task or remind you of the task if you start to get busy and are likely to forget it. Setting a reminder will draw you out of your hyperfocused state as well, so you don't spend too long on any one activity.

With a plan in place, you'll both feel more equipped to take on missteps as they happen. Of course, you probably won't always get it right, but things will run much more smoothly than they have been. Navigating the difficulties of the disorder can feel like a game of chance, but by using these tips and techniques, life is guaranteed to be much less stressful for you both.

When you've started to notice a change in the way things are running, you might be ready to spend more time together reconnecting and building intimacy. The non-affected partner will feel less burdened and less like a parent to the ADHD-affected partner. The affected partner will feel like they are accepted and wanted by the person they married. It's a win for everyone involved.

Chapter Summary

- ADHD symptoms can affect your relationship in many ways. Some of the most common symptoms that affect the relationship involve struggles with time management, organization, impulsive behavior, and emotional dysregulation.
- Both of you have a lot of feelings and emotions that the other might not understand or be aware of. It will help to take a step back and express how you're both feeling to better understand what the other is going through.
- For the non-affected spouse, remember to be patient, focus on their intentions, use positive reinforcement, and stop acting like their parent.
- For the affected spouse, it's important to acknowledge your role in the situation, take a step back when emotions run high, and build your resource toolbox for managing your symptoms.

- For both of you, remember to identify your emotions, set aside time for each other or just relax, put yourself in the other's shoes and go to counseling to help you talk through things you're still struggling with.
- There are a lot of unconventional ways you can work through your issues as well, such as participating in exercise together, finding humor in the absurd, and educating yourself more about ADHD.
- Put a plan in place for how you're going to improve things moving forward. Outsource and delegate tasks to lighten the load, act as a team and set up reminders, schedule weekly check-ins to see how things are going, and discuss concerns and develop a daily routine to help things run more smoothly.

In the next chapter, we're going to discuss overcoming anxieties in the relationship. We'll take a closer look at the ways you and your partner might be feeling distant from each other and how to bridge that gap.

Day Two: Overcome Relationship Anxieties

Exercise: Pick a room where you spend a lot of time together, like the bedroom. Sit together, facing each other. Take ten deep breaths, in for four, hold for four, out for six.

Reach out and hold each other's hands. Close your eyes and focus on the sensation of what you're feeling. Focus on the way you feel connected through your hands. Focus until the only thing you're aware of is the sound of their breathing and the feeling of their skin on yours.

Move your hands to each part of your partner's body in turn. Start with their hands and move in this order: hands, arms, shoulders, face, hair, chest, abdomen, thighs, lower legs, feet, back up to the thighs, and then optionally, onto your partner's sexual organs. Continue to meditate on each part in turn.

The purpose of this exercise is to feel more deeply connected and attuned to each other's bodies.

ADHD definitely affects your partner regarding relationship anxieties, but how do you experience anxiety? People with this disorder are more likely to suffer from comorbidities like depression, anxiety, and disordered behavior than their neurotypical counterparts. Anxiety can be a built-in part of the experience for many. It can feel all-consuming, with intrusive thoughts that plague you about the future and your lives together. Fear of the unknown can make you act rashly or badly in situations where understanding is needed.

Relationship anxieties are usually related to past experiences and trauma and, left unchecked, can poison even the healthiest of partnerships. Anxiety is like a wound that, left untreated, can end up destroying the body. Some of the worst anxieties that affected people face can add to the stress of relationships. For example, your partner may have impulsive behaviors that lead you to worry about the state of your finances. Impulsive behaviors and addictive tendencies are common. Your partner may be addicted to playing video games, spending too much money, or even having a more serious addiction to drugs or alcohol. It can be worrisome when they have an addictive personality, wondering what to do about their addiction and how to cope. You might also be feeling like you come second to your partner's special interests, and you feel like your partner doesn't listen when you tell them about your day or how you're feeling.

The difficulties with inattention might be making you feel ignored. Suppose your partner is constantly forgetting the things you say or forgetting important anniversaries, or not stepping up and showing their appreciation in ways that are meaningful to you. In that case, you might even start to wonder if they care. You could also feel like your partner expects you to perfectly manage them and their symptoms–that you need to be the "strong" one, the one in complete control who reminds them what they forgot or helps them when they have strong ADHD-powered emotions. You feel stressed at the thought that you're not always capable of meeting those needs.

For the affected partner, it can be all the same anxieties as the non-affected spouse and more. You probably spend a lot of time stressing about the future and what might happen instead of allowing yourself to be present and in the present in the relationship. People with ADHD often rush into relationships, craving the high of new love and then worrying about being "good enough" to sustain it. Additionally, you may experience a lot of anxiety revolving around your own negative qualities and how they're affecting the relationship. Due to a combination of poor self-esteem and past trauma, you could be assuming that a breakup is inevitable. You analyze every interaction and pick it apart for signs.

159

For people with the disorder, you could have had unfulfilling or bad past relationships, and you worry that the same problems will crop up again. You obsess over not repeating those mistakes, or you feel like you can't get a handle on the issues that led to the demise of your current relationship. Being socially adept is challenging for anyone but especially for people with this disorder. It might be stressful trying to decipher your partner's body language and decide whether or not they're upset with you. You are stressed about inadvertently or unintentionally embarrassing your partner in social situations. It can feel like you have to be careful about everything you say and do, especially if you had an overbearing parent about your social shortcomings.

When something goes wrong, you or your partner may place a lot of the blame on your symptoms. This can lead to you stressing over the idea that the relationship issues are your fault. You internalize the message. Instead of thinking, "this is from one of my symptoms," you tell yourself, "I am a terrible person causing issues."

Of course, this is just a snapshot of the types of anxieties that each spouse may be facing. The list is endless. Anxiety, like depression, likes to feed off of itself to remain a constant in the life of its host. The two of you may not even realize how many anxieties you have in common. Sharing those anxieties is the first step to overcoming them. Here are some ways you can better manage anxiety in relationships:

1. **Practice mindfulness**. Mindfulness is learning to be fully present and aware of what you're feeling and experiencing and doing in a non-judgmental, accepting way. There are many ways to practice mindfulness, from checking in with yourself every few hours to using meditation to center yourself and focus on your thoughts and feelings. Both of you need to spend time

160

centering yourself and understanding what you're feeling, where you're feeling it in your body, and why you feel the way you do. Mindfulness can help with that. As you become more aware of your feelings, you'll know how to combat negative thoughts.

2. **Practice breathing**. When you're feeling anxious or panicky or upset, taking a moment to breathe can make all the difference. Try different breathing techniques for calming yourself and bringing yourself back to a neutral state. Taking a step away during a disagreement to focus on your breathing can also be helpful, not only to quell anxieties but to re-center yourself.

3. **Challenge your fear.** Whenever a fear or anxiety crops up, face it head-on. Explain to yourself why the fear is unfounded. If you worry your partner will leave you, look at your wedding photos to remind yourself that they're committed to you for better or worse. If you fear that the house will never get spotless, remind yourself that it doesn't have to be perfect, just clean *enough*. A little dust on the baseboards never killed anyone. You can always sit down and discuss your fears with your partner as well. Your partner may be more reassuring than you expect and less judgmental than you fear.

4. **Identify your triggers**. If certain things or situations trigger your anxieties, identify those. You can help your spouse by avoiding those things that upset them or finding ways to help them when those pop up. For example, if new social situations trigger your spouse's ADHD, stick with them to help them navigate a new situation. Leaving them to fend for themselves isn't fair or kind. As the non-ADHD spouse, if you are

highly bothered by clothes all over the bedroom floor, set a timer for 15 minutes where the two of you clean up all the clothes, putting them away or in the laundry. Working together can help you both feel more like a team.

5. **Practice socializing**. It can be incredibly stressful to navigate social situations, especially for people with ADHD. Practice socializing either with your spouse or a counselor. You can go over situations and how to handle them and any kind of issues that crop up for you. For example, maybe you talk over people too much while socializing. Practice using small cues like a tap on the wrist with your spouse that they can use when you're dominating the conversation. You'll feel more confident that you can enjoy social situations without being off-putting.

6. **Have a safeword**. Sometimes when things get overwhelming, you just need an out. Use a safeword like "sunshine" or "Carole Baskin" to let your spouse know that you're experiencing anxiety in a situation. It doesn't matter if you're around other people or you're using it in private, using your safeword should mean that your spouse knows you need comforting. The non-affected spouse should aim to make the affected spouse as comfortable as possible, either removing them from the situation or ending the discussion until further notice.

7. **Commit to commitment**. As people affected, we often crave excitement and new situations. This can easily lead to feeling the urge to stray. When this happens, you should talk to your spouse, first and foremost, and definitely seek therapy. In addition to that, find ways to spice things up with your spouse.

Pick something exciting to look forward to doing together. This can be as simple as a new movie you both want to see or as wild as trying new sexual positions on an exotic vacation. The important thing is to focus on staying committed to your spouse.

8. **Forgive and forget**. Holding grudges or holding onto all the ways you two have messed up over the years is not only toxic for your relationship, but it can easily destroy your self-esteem. Learn to let go of your anger and frustration and forgive your partner for their mistakes. You also have to learn to let it go and no longer bring up past transgressions. It will be much healthier in the long run. You're spending a lifetime together, petty grudges have no place here.

9. **Only one crazy person in the house at a time**. Make it a rule that when one of you is freaking out or having a panic attack, the other has to be calm and collected. Only one person is allowed to go nuts at any given time. It's a silly but effective rule.

10. **Find ways to connect**. When you have anxieties over the state of the relationship, take time to connect. Play a video game together, pick a tv show to binge-watch on your favorite streaming service, or do an activity together like taking a walk or completing a puzzle. The simple act of doing something together will be reassuring and comforting. You'll feel more connected to each other when you spend quality time together. It can be hard to find the time in this busy world but schedule it out if needed. Set aside one hour a week where the two of you sit down or get out and do something together.

11. **Seek help**. Sometimes you need more help than a few breathing exercises can provide. Whether you go to a

counselor or see your healthcare provider for medication, find a way to manage the anxiety that works for you. There's no shame in needing the extra help. Sometimes, fighting depression and anxiety can feel like fighting a war. You can't win a war if you're not properly prepared. Medication can be like the armor that protects you during battle. It's armor that you can use to get through. However, you can't win a war without proper assistance. You need fellow soldiers and leaders who can guide you through. Mental health specialists can be like your leaders, while your friends and family can be your fellow fighters. Once properly prepared to fight, there's no way you can lose.

Anxiety can easily get the best of us. Sometimes, it can get so bad that it destroys the relationship. When this happens, you need to take a serious step back and reach for help. Some of the most damaging behaviors to relationships stem from anxiety. Be on the lookout for behaviors that show that your partner lets their anxieties control them in damaging ways. Your partner has the right to a certain degree of say in a relationship, but you also have a right to decide what that level of control looks like. It's an issue when they begin to decide things for you that you don't agree with or feel uncomfortable about. Anxiety can drive people to control their partner's actions in fear of what might happen to them if they don't take control. This is unfair and infantilizing to your adult spouse. Try to realize that your partner is their own person with their own mind, and they deserve to be treated like an adult. Being constantly interrogated about where you're going or who you're with can feel stifling. Does your partner accuse you of things baselessly? Be aware of this red flag. Your partner might be coming from a place of anxiety and poor self-esteem, maybe feeling like they're in a relationship with someone "out of their league" or "too good for them," but ultimately, that's a problem for them to fix. Try to nip it in the bud as quickly as possible when this crops up.

Jealousy can stem from a multitude of places that are all rooted in insecurity and anxiety. It's easy to get swallowed up by the green-eyed monster when you feel like your spouse is more successful or more adept than you. Instead of becoming infected with jealousy, focus on the fact that the two of you are a team, and their success is your success. Sometimes, the affected spouse might feel like their relationship has become dull, lopsided, or unfulfilling and seek advice and comfort elsewhere. This is emotional cheating. Find a way to address the issue that has led to impulsive behaviors and fix it.

The non-affected spouse might have reached a point where they begin to resent every moment with the affected spouse. They begin to belittle them or criticize them unfairly, nitpicking every little thing until the affected spouse feels torn to pieces. Contempt for your partner can demoralize them and make them less likely to want to open up to you when things are wrong. Avoid this behavior at all costs. If you feel resentful, try to remind yourself of their good qualities. Do it every day if necessary. The affected spouse might feel tired of being criticized or nagged, and you begin to stonewall yourself to end the seemingly constant criticism. You refuse to engage, and you no longer want to listen to what they have to say, so you put up a cold front. It may be hard to hear their criticism, but the best way to address that is to communicate instead of refusing to engage. You are inadvertently telling your spouse that you don't care what they have to say when you do this.

You might be tempted to shut down and disengage from the world when anxiety runs high. You feel as though it's safer and you can protect yourself by not caring at all. In reality, you're coming across as apathetic to your spouse. They may begin to feel like you don't care, or you're falling out of love, or that they love you more than you love them. Instead of shutting out the entire world, let your spouse in when things are bad. It can be tempting to run away from your problems. You think you'll feel better after running away, but the problems you left behind aren't going anywhere. All you're doing is upsetting your spouse more and avoiding responsibility. It can feel tough to own up to your problems and admit to your mistakes, but it's healthier for your mental well-being and your relationship.

These behaviors can certainly be damaging to the relationship. They can be downright destructive if left unchecked. If your partner does any of these and you feel like they aren't changing, you should seek therapy. Things can change, but only if both partners are willing to put the work in and the effort.

Some of the best ways to manage if one or both of you are affected by anxiety is to seek therapy or counseling to manage your issues. Mental health care has a stigma because many people believe that it's only for "crazy" people or insist that they are too private to talk about things. It might be hard to encourage someone to seek therapy who is resistant. This can stall the progress in a relationship and cause negative feelings and resentment. You need to be sensitive to the other person's mental state and the timing of your discussion. You don't want to start the discussion in front of other people, potentially embarrassing or upsetting them. You also want to be careful not to blurt it out in the middle of an argument or while they've been highly stressed or in a bad mood. They may get defensive and refuse to engage further because they believe they're being labeled. Also, a group-style intervention will simply anger them and make them put up more walls. They may not be comfortable with others knowing or interfering in their problems. Be mindful of choosing a time when they are relaxed, and you're alone. *Tip*: Ask them if they're in a good headspace for you to offer a suggestion. You already know if your loved one is open to the idea of help. You should prepare for a no, or repeatedly hearing no. Start by pointing out their good qualities;

166

you're more likely to appeal to someone who is resistant. You can remind them that they're more than their issues. They don't have to be defined by their mistakes. It gives them a chance to see that working on their issues is just that–working on issues. Make sure they know how important your relationship is with them. They may be more likely to understand that you want to improve the relationship or avoid further damage. Be wary of using ultimatums, though. Get specific about the areas you want to see changes. When people refuse therapy, they may believe they don't have a problem. Avoid being judgmental but let them know the areas that you see could use improvement.

They may be aware they need help but are afraid to seek it because of the stigma around mental health support. Using non-stigmatizing language to support them through their journey can be a way to encourage them. Here are some examples of phrases and words to use and to avoid when speaking to your partner:

- **Do not use:** *Psycho.* "You're so psycho about this." This can make your loved one feel judged and angry.
- **Do not use:** *Crazy.* "You're acting crazy right now!" Crazy, like psycho, makes people more likely to avoid seeking help if they believe they're being labeled.
- **Do not use**: *Paranoid.* "I can't believe how paranoid you're acting." This may make your loved one feel as though *you* think they're overreacting.
- **Do use:** *I will support you. I'm there for you. You can do this.*
- **Do use:** *You are facing difficulties. You seem to be going through a tough time.*
- **Do use:** *You seem to be mistrustful/fearful right now.*

Sometimes they might not know where to start, or it might feel overwhelming to figure out how to set it up. They might be hesitant about seeing a therapist on their own or exposing their issues in a group session. You can offer to go with them for the first few sessions or sit in the waiting room while they're there. You can ensure them that whatever they talk about in therapy is private, and you won't pry for information. They need to feel that they can work through their issues in a safe, non-confrontational manner. If you're there expecting to hear all about it afterward, they may not want to go for fear of being pushed to talk about something they can barely talk about themselves. Make sure that any information they share with you about their therapy session stays private. Sometimes it's tempting to discuss the issue with a close friend or family member, but if they think you're telling their business, they will be even more reluctant to go.

Going to therapy can be a big deal for many. Ensure you're supportive if they decide they're ready to seek help. Be positive and encouraging, and reinforce their decision with positive affirmations. Reassure them of your love throughout the process. Above all, be patient with them and with yourself. Celebrate your victories together and let go of judgment.

Of course, you and your partner can work on issues together. You can seek therapy to help yourself with areas that need improvement, but what can you do on your own to help minimize your own relationship anxieties? Start with making sure you're practicing self-care. Self-care is a hot buzzword these days, but it just means you need to ensure you put your own oxygen mask on first. Before you can work on relationship issues or help your spouse with their issues, you need to look at yourself and examine how you can help yourself feel safe, happy, and cared for. Next, communicate your needs. It might feel like simplistic advice, but are you truly communicating what you need to your partner? It's possible you're bottling it up or expecting them to be a mind reader. Misunderstandings and anger can be avoided when you are clear with what you need. The uncertainties that cause anxiety can then be eliminated.

One of the biggest sources of anxiety is a fear of the future. You fear not having certainty or stress about things that have yet to happen. Take a step back and try to enjoy the present moment in your relationship. There will always be things to worry about, but you can't spend every second worrying or you'll never enjoy the relationship. Whether you have trauma from a past relationship or worry about being good enough, looking internally at your anxieties can help you discover where they may be coming from. What is causing your stress and worry? How can you manage those anxieties to lessen stress in your current relationship? If you're not doing something to manage the stress and anxieties, you're letting them pile up until you explode on each other. It's important to remember that the two of you are a team and that it's okay to bring your anxieties and stresses to each other to help you cope. You'd be surprised at how your spouse may come up with solutions for problems that you didn't even think of—as part of their ability to think outside the box.

Exercises for couples to manage anxieties

Even if you're not on the brink of divorce, here are a few ways you can come together to connect as a couple that will help your marriage:

- **Exercise One: Write a letter**. Write a romantic letter to your partner that focuses on the positive aspects of your relationship, such as the things that first attracted you or some of your favorite memories. Transition to discussing potential areas for growth near the end. Each of you will then silently read your partner's letter before discussing what you wrote about. This is a helpful way to express to your partner what works and what you like about the relationship while also getting across what you would like to work on.

- **Exercise Two: Emotional check-ins**. Choose three emotions you experienced that day to share. The other partner should reflect on your emotions. Example: "It sounds like you were tired, frustrated, and stressed today." Let your partner share the story behind those emotions. Giving your partner the space to express themselves gives you an idea of how to support your partner in whatever they're going through and give them emotional validation. They will feel supported and heard.
- **Exercise Three: Give daily affirmations.**Take time in the day to share two or three things you appreciate about the other person, even small things. Example: "I appreciate that you made me lunch, and I appreciate that you texted me during your break." Positive affirmations will work as positive reinforcement, and it builds trust and respect between the two of you.
- **Exercise Four: Breathe together.** Sit back-to-back in a comfortable position. Start by focusing on your breathing and notice the movement of your body. Then notice the movement of your spouse's body, focusing on them. Bring your breathing in sync for a few minutes. End with a hug. You're working on being more in sync with this exercise and practicing mindfulness.
- **Exercise Five: Watch romantic shows and movies**. Research shows that couples who watch movies together and discuss them afterward for approximately 45 minutes show improvement akin to couples who go to therapy together. This is because it gives you the practice of communicating about relationship issues in a very low-stakes way. Romantic movies are best as they focus on relationships between couples.

- **Exercise Six: Create a wishlist**. Take turns writing down three or more things you'd like more of or less of in the relationship. Use "I" statements to express your desires and how you would feel if the wishes came true. The wishlist is an exercise that allows the two of you to express your needs while in a calm headspace. You and your partner can also visualize what the relationship could look like if the change occurs.

- **Exercise Seven: "The story I'm telling myself."** This exercise is beneficial when you're in the midst of a conflict and projecting your insecurities onto your partner. For example, instead of being accusatory, i.e. "You spend too much time going out with your friends!" you might say, "The story I'm telling myself is that you'd rather spend time with your friends than with me because I'm annoying you." This can frame your feelings in a way that takes ownership of your feelings and your perception of the situation without casting blame on your partner. This gives your partner the chance to share their side of their story, and you two can work things out together.

Chapter Summary

- Relationship anxieties stem from both partners feeling as if their wants and needs aren't met for whatever reason.
- For the affected partner, it may be due to the symptoms of their disorder that cause them to feel fearful, inadequate or misunderstand things. For the non-affected partner, they may be lonely and stressed from accommodating their partner's needs and feel as if their own aren't met.

- Insecurities, if left unchecked, can lead to downright hurtful behaviors, such as being controlling, contempt, emotional affairs, apathy, and running away.
- Take steps to beat insecurities by finding ways to connect with your partner, such as ensuring you're communicating your needs, watching romantic movies together, practicing mindfulness, and owning up to your insecurities. Therapy is also a great option to work through those issues together or separately.

In the next chapter, we will look at some of the relationship issues that come up, including how to build better social skills and tips for couples to understand each other better, including their nonverbal cues.

Day Three: Improve Relationship Skills

Exercise: Stand or sit comfortably, try to relax, and focus on your breathing. Keep your eyes open. Pick something around you that you enjoy looking at, and keep your gaze focused on that item.

Your thoughts may wander, but let them. The less you worry about your wandering thoughts, the easier it will be for them to leave independently. Keep returning your gaze to the object. Continually try to focus on the object in your vision. You're creating a mindful focus. Try this exercise when you're waiting, such as in traffic or stuck in a long line.

Those with the disorder may struggle with their social skills and managing when it comes to social interaction. They may have underdeveloped interpersonal communication skills and a poor understanding of navigating social situations. As a result,they may come across as abrasive, hurtful, scatterbrained, aggressive, overly emotional, too sensitive, or outright disruptive in social settings. This can interfere not only with the relationship between the two of you but your interpersonal relationships as a couple as well. Their interactions with others may be filled with miscommunications and misunderstandings. It can be stressful when, for example, a parent is uncomfortable letting their child have a playdate with your child because of your spouse. Or, it can be difficult to navigate when your spouse accidentally offends your family at dinner.

ADHD has many effects on the way that people navigate the world and how they understand it. They cannot understand social cues. They may zone out during conversations, and they end up missing important details or agreeing to something that they didn't realize as a result. Forgetfulness can mean that they don't get things done that you expect. Poor organizational skills can make you feel frustrated at the state of how messy the house gets or how disorganized your important paperwork becomes. Their emotional outbursts can hurt your feelings and make you feel like you have to walk on eggshells to avoid their temper. They are also more likely to give in to impulsivity which can mean blurting out inappropriate comments or engaging in reckless or irresponsible behavior.

As the non-affected partner, you have your own difficulties in navigating the relationship between ADHD and your partner. Are you constantly shooting them pointed looks when they speak? Do you criticize them for every small misstep or misspoken word? You could be causing more anxiety in your partner than you realize. Often we observe our spouse's interactions through a filtered lens rather than objectively. Was that joking comment really upsetting, or are you on the lookout for your partner offending people because of past behavior? It's possible you're too ready to jump to everyone else's defense instead of taking a step back and letting your partner navigate the world on their own.

Social skills get developed in childhood and adolescence. Children play pretend to understand the world around them. They copy adults or peers, observe situations, practice, and get feedback to acquire their skills. "They may pick up bits and pieces of what is appropriate but lack an overall view of social expectations. Unfortunately, as adults, they often realize "something" is missing but are never quite sure what that 'something' may be" (CHADD, n.d.). As a result, they may struggle with social acceptance. Peers may have viewed or labeled them as "weird" or pushed them into outcast status growing up. They may have been stuck outside the peer groups which would have led to better development of social skills.

There are many ways in which the disorder can affect a person's ability to navigate social situations and enjoy positive social interactions. The symptoms often hinder one's ability to understand and navigate situations in several key areas. Here are the common challenges most people with ADHD face when it comes to social skills:

- **Challenge #1: Inability to pick up on social cues.** Does it ever feel like everyone around you is in on some kind of joke that you just don't get? Do you feel like you frequently break "unspoken" social rules? It can be challenging to navigate in social situations when your social meter seems broken. For example, you miss out when someone's raised eyebrow indicates that they find your comment in poor taste or accidentally keep interrupting someone trying to tell a story.

  How you can work together: Help your spouse with subtle cues when they're talking over people. Be there to explain jokes they may not understand or reassure them when someone is teasing or being sarcastic.

- **Challenge #2: Trouble keeping friendships.** Some people may experience you as too intense or needy. You are coming across as demanding of their time and attention without realizing it. It can feel like your friendships flame quickly and fizzle out quickly. Do you feel like you have a lot of great connections that don't end up going anywhere? Your symptoms may be causing you to alienate people without realizing it.

  How you can work together: Join a team sport or league together. You'll be there to keep an eye on your spouse while still giving them the space to make their

175

own friendships. This also gets the two of you active and out of the house. Physical activity can be a great way to help manage symptoms of ADHD so it will be easier for your spouse to feel in control in a setting like this because they won't be as stressed about managing their emotions–the exercise will give them the boost they need.

- **Challenge #3: Overreacting.** With ADHD, it can be difficult to control your emotions. There is an impairment in the brain that means the brain itself can't properly regulate your emotional reactions to situations. You end up "overreacting" to something someone has said or done. You have meltdowns when things aren't going well. This can feel offputting to people who don't understand you.

  How you can work together: Talk through the things that push your anger buttons the most. Identify how it feels when your anger is reaching critical mass. Then, work on finding ways to mitigate the situation when it's getting to the point of no return.

- **Challenge #4: Being scatterbrained and "unreliable."** One of the symptoms of ADHD is the inability to focus on the information being presented. You also have trouble with planning tasks and following through. These can lead to people feeling as though you're unreliable to them and that you can't be counted on when it's important.

  How you can work together: Keep track of the things people have asked of your partner together. Have them write everything down, and the two of you can go over the tasks in the evening to plan out how your spouse will tackle them or how the two of you can work on them together.

Affected adults may struggle with making and keeping friendships and be labeled as "difficult" or "problematic" in work settings or adult peer groups. There is an impairment in the executive functioning of the brain, and, as a result, it may feel impossible to learn the skills that everyone else seems to find innate. It's not an impossible task, however. There are ways to learn to create better social skills that will help both of you. To understand subtext, look for context clues. Observe what people are saying and be aware that their words may have alternative meanings. "We can do it when I'm less busy!" might mean "I'd love to when I have less on my plate." It might also mean "I'm politely brushing you off." Be aware of their body language, tone of voice, or the look in their eyes for clues as to what they might be saying. Spend time observing the choice of words someone uses to understand the meaning behind their words better. If they say, "I would love to go!" that probably means they want to go. "If you want to" might mean it's a reluctant yes or a polite no. Consider the phrase "actions speak louder than words." If they say one thing and do another, it would be smart to consider how their actions reveal their true feelings.

When all else fails, use your spouse as a guide. With your spouse's help, the two of you can work on the way you understand those around you. Ask how their interpretation of a situation compares with your interpretation. This is helpful when you feel like you're constantly getting things wrong. Also, be aware that polite behaviors usually disguise people's real feelings. We have created a society that values being polite over being honest, and oftentimes, people choose to spare your feelings instead of saying how they really feel. To decode them better, observe them. Watch how other people in a social setting are acting or behaving. Look at Pinterest or Google for ideas of how to dress or what to wear in certain social occasions. Be deferent

177

to different cultures and customs. Don't be afraid to ask for help if you're stumped.

When you get really excited, you might be speaking too quickly for others to keep up or get a word edgewise. Slow down and take a deep breath so that people around you can participate in the conversation. You can still share your excitement or passion for a topic but give people room to join in. Another way to help yourself deal with your anxieties in social situations is to add a fidget toy or object that you can play with to help decrease anxiety and excess energy. Sitting still might be hard in a formal setting such as a lecture or theater performance, but a non-distracting fidget toy can give you an outlet. Additionally, before a social event, get out excess energy by doing some light exercise or taking a short walk can burn off excess energy before you leave.

If you feel like you're missing information, look your companions in the eye or set down whatever you're doing to give them your full attention. It might be tempting to send a quick work email while you're on the phone with your friend or text your partner a funny meme while having a long conversation with your mom but these actions can come across as disrespectful because you're ignoring them and missing relevant information. Additionally, consider a social skills coach. There are life coaches and therapists who specialize in helping people build up their social skills. Get in touch with someone you think can help and find a strategy together to work through your most troubling situations.

When it comes to understanding nonverbal communication, people with ADHD definitely have a disadvantage. Still, it's possible the non-affected spouse might also be struggling to understand their partner's nonverbal communication. Both partners give off cues with body language, tone, eye contact, etc. that the other might not be picking up on. This can be damaging to the relationship for both parties. When trying to communicate, you can work on being more open with each other about your feelings, and you can speak to a therapist about what you're struggling to speak about, but it's a whole different story to pick up on the things your partner *isn't* saying.

These are the types of nonverbal communication cues that your partner may be expressing:

- **Facial expression**. Fun fact: The facial expressions for many emotions are the same across almost all cultures. Happiness, anger, sadness, surprise, fear, and disgust are universal. Your face can make many expressions and indicate many kinds of emotions.
- **Body movement and posture**. Your posture can indicate many things, such as pride, annoyance, fatigue, or contempt. People show how they feel in how they walk, stand, sit and hold their heads.
- **Gestures**. People use gestures to communicate many things. You can wave hello or point to show a location. You make an okay sign to indicate agreement or put a palm up to say "stop!" Some gestures that are acceptable in one country might be considered offensive in another. For example, a peace sign facing the wrong way is a rude gesture in the United Kingdom. In some cultures, pointing a single finger is rude; using two fingers is a better way to communicate.
- **Eye contact**. Eye contact is one of the first ways we communicate with others. There's a saying that the eyes are the window to the soul, and your eyes can indicate the way you feel even when the rest of you might be hiding your feelings. Some people find maintaining eye contact important during a conversation as a meter to measure interest and respect.

- **Touch**. We often measure our level of respect or closeness through touch. A firm handshake shows strength. A hug is sometimes uncomfortable if you're not close enough to the person you're touching. We even use touch to indicate our interest in someone. For example, a light touch on the arm can go a long way in flirting with another person.
- **Space**. People can be particular about their personal space. If you've ever been made uncomfortable by someone standing too close or getting into your space during a discussion, you understand how space can be used to communicate.
- **Voice**. More than the words spoken, messages can be communicated through how they are spoken. People can often tell sincerity in your tone of voice or sarcasm or contempt. You can communicate fondness or intimacy depending on how you raise or lower your voice.

The way you communicate using body language or nonverbal cues can affect how other people see and perceive you and how much they like or respect you. Based on nonverbal cues, they may even decide whether or not to trust you. If you've ever heard someone say, "I don't like that person's vibes." Or, "Something about that person makes me distrust them," it's nothing special or magical. It's more than likely due to the unconscious nonverbal signals they give off. When you send negative or confusing signals without intending to, communication can become muddled, and connection and trust become damaged.

Improving your ability to interpret nonverbal communication isn't hard; it's a skill that can be learned like anything else. You and your spouse should start by spending time observing each other throughout the day. How does their posture change when stressed or tired? What is it like when they're happy or excited? Does their tone change when speaking to you about chores?

For the affected spouse, this can be a helpful way to figure out how to understand others' nonverbal cues. For the non-affected spouse, you can start to pick up on nonverbal cues that indicate when your partner is struggling or losing attention or having trouble understanding you. Being more observant can make it easier to figure out how to adapt and change to better meet each other's needs. Don't be shy about expressing your affections. Smile at your spouse, look them in the eye, or reach out and touch them when the mood strikes. Hold their hand when you walk together and give them a hug or kiss when leaving. By showing how you feel without words, you increase your trust in each other.

Make sure you're giving them the attention they deserve. Pay attention to how your partner might feel through their nonverbal cues. Are they crossing their arms? They might be agitated. Are they sighing a lot? They may be sad or depressed. Trying to gain a sense of their feelings this way will help you better understand your partner and improve your communication skills with each other. Additionally, give each other surprise nonverbal affection such as a hug when they are talking to you about their day or hold their hand while you're watching a movie together. Surprises keep the romance alive.

If you observe your partner giving off nonverbal cues that you struggle to interpret, ask if what you're observing is correct. Try to avoid asking, "What's wrong?" and point out your observations. They'll appreciate that you're paying attention to their cues instead of expecting them always to explain themselves. When you're in a disagreement or argument, try to refrain from using negative nonverbal cues like eye-rolling and sighing. Put your phone away when your partner is talking to you. These will eliminate misunderstandings and help avoid escalation of conflict.

To improve your connection with each other, plan a weekly date night or have coffee together every morning. Pick something to do together that encourages you to connect with each other. Be happy to see each other. When you greet your spouse with warmth and seem genuinely excited to see each other, you're fostering a positive association with coming home.

If you're having problems understanding each other, seek out help from someone who understands relationship issues, like a relationship coach. They can help you learn how to communicate better and understand each other's nonverbal cues and communication. Nonverbal cues can be difficult to master, but with time and practice, you will feel yourself and your spouse learning how to navigate each other's communication much easier. It will even help with people outside of your family, with work, and your friendships. You struggle with maintaining relationships as a couple from the symptoms affecting your spouse. It's easy to blame your partner for "messing up" the relationship, but are you working together effectively to navigate social situations? Are you helping your spouse, or are you waiting until they make a mistake and then berating them about it later? It might feel like waiting to talk to them is the best or the only way to get through to them, but there are actually better techniques the two of you can utilize.

If one or both of you are struggling with your social and interpersonal communication skills, there are ways the two of you can work together to make navigating life as a couple much easier. Helping each other through the difficulties is one of the pillars of a healthy relationship. When you work together, you reinforce that you're a team. Before you go into a social situation, know that one of you might want to leave before the other is ready. Agree on a time that works for the both of you and have a strategy for when it's time to go that saves you both from any stress or embarassment. Also, make sure you're planning ahead. When you know something is coming up, plan for all eventualities, like forgetting things, running late, ADHD triggers, etc. Having a plan to deal with eventualities will help you both feel more confident.

If you know certain situations highly upset you, try to find a way to avoid them or ways to deal with them. If you're getting tired from socialization, take a break or go somewhere quiet. If you're struggling with ADHD symptoms, step away for a while. If your partner needs to step away for their sanity, don't assume they're abandoning you. If the non-affected partner gently and quietly corrects you, don't assume they're trying to embarrass you. Give each other the benefit of the doubt. Find the quiet areas together that can offer a place for retreat.

Knowing what to say in social situations can be extremely helpful. Prepare scripts ahead of time that you can use to answer common questions that come up or appropriate responses to small talk. Practice small talk with your partner to feel more comfortable. When one of you is having a difficult time or needs space, make sure that the other is covering for you or running interference to help you out. Collaborate as partners to figure out how you can help each other best.

It's also better to navigate social situations by figuring out your priorities. Come together to discuss what your priorities as a couple are. What social situations are necessary, and what is less important? What situations are necessary to navigate as a couple, and what situations can handle just one of you attending?

When things go wrong, develop a code word or gesture that helps out in awkward, uncomfortable, or triggering situations. Use that to quietly indicate when you need help, or you can tell your partner is getting overstimulated. Check in with each other every few hours. If you have an agreed-upon time to leave, check-in within a half-hour and ask your partner if they're still comfortable leaving at the agreed-upon time or if they'd like to stay. Check and make sure they are comfortable and enjoying themselves. Ask and make sure that everything is still going alright. Don't forget also to be aware of any triggers. It can be easy to enter a situation, expecting things to go well, only for an unexpected trigger to pop up. Knowing your partner's triggers ahead of time can help you both navigate when it happens.

It can often feel overwhelming for people with the disorder to navigate new social situations, especially if socialization is important for your partner. Rather than making them go to new events, meet new people, and try new things every week, do one new thing a month or let them spend a limited amount of time socializing while building up their tolerance. Try to push yourself outside your comfort zone from time to time. Even if it feels difficult, sometimes your partner needs to accompany them into a situation you aren't comfortable with. You don't have to do it every day, or even every week, but find activities that are a little out of your comfort zone. Learn about your partner's special interests or as the affected partner, go with them to their college reunion. You two should also ensure that you both have alone time. You both need time to be alone and recharge. Make sure you schedule a time for yourselves each day or each week. Having time to recharge can help when you come back together. You will then feel refreshed and ready to reconnect.

Lastly, there are probably things that you are just more comfortable dealing with than your spouse. For example, one of you might not mind calling the doctor to schedule appointments or taking the food from the delivery driver. One of you might be better at asking for playdates for your children from fellow parents or talking to the school administration. Pick tasks that you can handle and trade for the harder ones for you. These tips will help the two of you navigate the situations that occur when living life as a couple. It's never bad to practice socializing and have contingency plans for when things go awry. Continue working with a therapist for more difficult situations, though.

Consider the following scenarios and how you would use the above tips as a couple to effectively manage what happens:

Scenario #1: Carlos and Andrew are set to attend a weekly family dinner together. Carlos' family is very loving and accepting of their son-in-law, but Andrew, who has ADHD, feels anxious about spending another dinner with Carlos' family. They usually arrive around 5 p.m., but Andrew gets tired of social interaction quickly, and the family typically doesn't start eating dinner until much later in the evening. They are also quick to joke and rib each other. Andrew feels left out because he doesn't always get the jokes. Sometimes, when he jokes back, his jokes don't match Carlos' family's sense of humor and they fall flat or offend the person on the receiving end. Andrew doesn't want to go, but Carlos insists, as it's an important family tradition to have dinner together every Sunday. How would the two of you work together to navigate this dynamic?

Scenario #2: Zahra and Eli are parents to Moses, who is in the third grade. Eli is a social butterfly and often arranges playdates for their son with family friends' children. Eli has been busy lately, and their son has asked mom to arrange a playdate with his best friend Zolan. Mom has ADHD and the thought of calling up Zolan's mom gives her anxiety as she and Abby don't get along. She doesn't know why Abby has a problem with her, but it affects her son's relationship with his best friend. Mom wants dad to do it, but he's about to leave to travel abroad for work and doesn't really have time. Dad wants mom to feel more comfortable arranging playdates and interacting with other parents. How would the two of you handle this?

Scenario #3: Michael and Sophia are newlyweds. Michael has ADHD and has made it clear that he's not very open to new things.

185

He's got a few foods that he likes; he's got a few places in town that he enjoys going to visit, but he mostly stays at home and keeps to himself. Sophia doesn't want to change him, but she does want to try new things here and there. She begs Michael to try a new Indian restaurant that's opened just down the street. Michael reluctantly agrees but ends up not enjoying himself. Sophia is mad that Michael now refuses to try any new restaurants or bars. She ends up going out herself almost every weekend with her friends, while Michael stays at home, lonely without his new wife. How would the two of you handle this situation?

There is no one right answer to each of the scenarios. The answers depend on the shared values and priorities that you have. How you make the situations work is entirely up to you. With each new situation you experience, each unique challenge, you have the opportunity to grow as a couple as you work together to navigate. Some days, it can feel like having ADHD means you don't get to live the lives of a couple that you imagined or that it's ruining your relationships–but you don't have to continue to feel that way anymore.

Chapter Summary

- Symptoms can interfere with your ability to navigate social situations, which can affect your social life. It can feel like your symptoms are getting the better of you, but there are ways to learn to improve and to mitigate when things go wrong.
- Build a social skills toolkit that helps you better understand others and things you can use when you're struggling. Examples include using context clues, looking to your spouse as a guide, and observing their nonverbal cues.

- Nonverbal cues can be particularly difficult for people with ADHD to navigate. Nonverbal cues include eye contact, body language, tone of voice, posture, and facial expressions.
- You can work together on gaining a better understanding of each other's nonverbal cues, which will help the both of you identify and manage when symptoms are becoming an issue.
- Have a plan for potential problems and ways you'll work together to solve them when going into a social situation. Plan an exit strategy, run interference, and find ways to avoid your triggers or get away to a quiet space.

In the next chapter, we'll look at conflicts for affected couples and how to navigate them and resolve them in positive, healthy ways.

Day Four: Resolve Conflicts in a Healthy Way

Exercise: Try this when you're both in the midst of an argument and need a break from the discussion. Take three steps apart from each other, breathe in for four, hold for four, our for six. Repeat three times in a row.

Next, step forward again until you're touching your palms. Let your thoughts go. Focus on the way your partner feels. Imagine what their emotions are at the moment. Try to connect with their body and their emotions. Let yourself focus on them, on their state of being. Do this for five to ten minutes, and then when you're done, resume the discussion.

Understanding how to manage when conflict arises is the cornerstone of any successful marriage. Knowing how to communicate in a healthy manner, how to compromise, how to handle disagreements, and even how to argue successfully are all vital to ensuring a happy life together. With the presence of the disorder though, it can become extremely difficult to manage when conflict arises. The affected partner may have difficulty articulating what is going wrong for them. The non-affected partner might feel as though they struggle to get through when communicating. There are definitely hurdles to get through in an ADHD-affected marriage. The key is to work within the symptoms and not against them.

Conflict exists in every relationship. No relationship is ever going to be one-hundred percent conflict-free. Even the best relationships may struggle with resolving conflict in a healthy manner. We can easily get stuck in a mindset that "I'm right and you're wrong," which doesn't bode well for a productive discussion. It's similar for people with the disorder as well. There is a disconnect for them in which it's difficult to process and understand the emotions and feelings of others. It may seem like they lack empathy, and it's true, to a degree. They also struggle to understand and process their own emotions as well, though. To better manage conflict, it's important to understand how and when conflict normally arises, how to be a good listener, how to argue effectively, and how to be a productive problem-solver.

Conflict arises when you and your partner strongly disagree with one another. The conflict may be unintentional on one partner's end, or one or both of you are unaware of the conflict. When situations arise that have us feeling a lot of emotion, we may be provoked or upset by others' reactions. However, no discussion is going to be productive if you cannot understand what your emotions are saying. You're putting the onus on your partner to fix things, and that's unfair to them. You could be unintentionally expecting your partner to be a mind reader because you can't understand what you're feeling but expect them to be able to resolve the conflict themselves.

Conflict can arise when one partner feels the other isn't being honest, when you disagree about values, or when you have strongly differing opinions. The things you two disagree on can range from values and beliefs such as whether or not to have children, how to raise them, how to manage finances, where you want to live, etc., to smaller decisions such as what to have for dinner, where to go on vacation, to trivial things like who fed the dog last or whose turn it is to empty the dishwasher. Conflict can be normal and good–such as when you're standing up for yourself in defense of your beliefs or against injustice–but it can also be problematic when conflict arises too often. Again, it's about learning to strike a balance for both of you.

When conflict arises, the first difficulty is often understanding where it's coming from. Discovering what causes conflict among you will help you understand yourself and each other better. For people with the disorder, their emotions can often become more intense and exaggerated. This is because there is an issue with the brain that prevents you from regulating intense emotions the same way that neurotypical people can. You literally cannot control how intense the emotions feel. You're also extremely sensitive to criticism and disapproval. This is often called Rejection Sensitive Dysphoria (RSD), which can cause symptoms similar to anxiety and depression when faced with feeling rejected or criticized. What you can control, though, is how you work through those intense emotions at the moment. Sometimes you need to take a step back before you blow up at your partner or lash out to hurt them.

One way to do that is to keep a journal where you write down your feelings. By journaling, you can begin to understand yourself better. For example, you'll be able to understand why you were so upset when you heard slight uncertainty in your spouse's tone when you suggested pizza for dinner or why you were so upset when they criticized how you loaded the dishwasher. You might also want to take space during the heat of the moment. You'll avoid lashing out in anger and defensiveness if you walk away. You may feel like your anger is making you want to explode and walking away can allow you to calm down and reassess the situation. You'll be able to come back to the discussion with a greater understanding and be able to work through things more calmly and rationally. It can definitely sting when our partner isn't excited about something we suggest, or we feel like they're being overly critical of the way we do things around the house.

As the non-affected spouse, you could also be unintentionally pushing their symptom triggers by the way you approach your critiques. If you're trying to comment on something, it might sound more like criticism, bringing up feelings of shame and defeat. If you're constantly questioning them because you don't trust their memory, you are probably pushing them to feel demoralized when they forget something. When you criticize them about their spending habits, they will feel as though they can't be trusted with a single cent without

190

being questioned. It's frustrating when your partner struggles with things that come easier to you, and it's easy to dismiss their symptoms as a failure on their part to step up. You ought to examine the way you approach them, though. Triggering their symptoms of shame, guilt, and anxiety will not correct the problem and will only damage the relationship over time.

If you come home and notice the dishes aren't done, despite asking, you use facts to guilt them, "The dishes aren't done." They are aware that they didn't complete the task asked. Or, if they genuinely forgot, they feel plenty of guilt without needing more, "I asked you to get the dishes done and you didn't listen." You nag them, repeatedly asking, "When are you going to do the dishes?" throughout the evening.

Instead of nagging, guilting, or shaming them, ask them "What would it take to get the dishes done?" People with the disorder often struggle with executive dysfunction, so a simple task like the dishes can feel inordinately overwhelming. For a neurotypical person, a task like doing the dishes might involve simply getting up and washing the dishes. For someone with ADHD, however, doing the dishes can be many steps, such as gathering the dishes around the house, ensuring there's enough soap, finding the sponges, putting away dishes from the dishwasher or drainer, soaking the plates with food residue, organizing the dishes into piles, etc. One task, in their minds, can feel like ten or more tasks. This doesn't even account for the fact that a task such as dishes involves standing still for a long time, which is one of the more difficult aspects of the disorder.

Recognizing the difficulty of approaching tasks is a helpful way to minimize conflict in the relationship. Once you're aware of how to work within the disorder's symptoms instead of against them, you'll discover that your spouse is more than capable of accomplishing anything you ask. One tip for dealing with an affected partner is to give them a to-do list. This is helpful as it gives them a visual reminder of the tasks required. It also eliminates the possibility of forgetting how verbal requests are often forgotten. Additionally, people with the disorder tend to enjoy checking off items on a to-do list. It gives them a boost of serotonin to visually see things getting done. Another tip is to help them out by sitting with them while they work. Body-doubling, as it's called, is a great way to help keep them focused. You can also help by working with them to help them break the task down into the steps needed so it feels less overwhelming.

It's also prudent to pick your battles. For example, if your partner cannot ever seem to remember to put their clothes in the hamper, but they're great at many other things, it might be time to let that battle go. It's not worth spending years of your life unhappy over something very minor. When you let go of the small things, your partner will also understand how important the big issues are to you. You'll also spend less time stressing yourself out. You'll gain more respect for your spouse as well. When you stop thinking of them as the enemy or focusing on all their little mistakes, you'll find yourself able to open your heart and fall in love with them all over again.

For times when it's harder to love your spouse or when you feel like their disorder is getting hard to separate from who they are as a person, you need to find a way to step back and reconnect. Start pointing out to yourself the things you like about them. Focus on the things you fell in love with. There will be days when you're stressed out because you're trying to juggle many plates in the air, and it feels like your spouse has let you down one time too many, but that's when it's most important to remind yourself of the good. Resentment builds where there is no love. If you're serious about making things work, you need to foster that love inside of you.

Another often unexplored cause of conflict between couples is the fact that people with the disorder often–consciously or unconsciously–create conflict as a way to get a boost of serotonin and dopamine. Their brains crave it and this stimulates the brain in ways that other things just can't. They may deny it, but it's not unheard of for a partner to look for ways to stir trouble. Again, this may not be a conscious thing on their part. "When the ADHD brain doesn't have enough stimulation, it looks for ways to increase its activity. Being angry or negative has an immediate stimulating effect on the brain." (Amen, 2020) There are a few ways that people with the disorder will engage their partner in drama games. One way they do this is by picking on others to get a rise out of them or upset them. Does your significant other pick something that upsets you to constantly tease you about, even after you've asked them to stop numerous times? Do you end up snapping or getting angry with them over that? You're giving their nervous system a shot of adrenaline, which raises your partner's heart rate and brain activity.

Another method they use is pushing your buttons to the point where you start yelling or screaming at them. People with the disorder can pick up your most vulnerable spots and target them. Being less reactive to this can even increase the behavior at first. They want to push and push until you explode. Some people with the disorder end up being more argumentative and oppositional. They get a rush from saying "no" to your request or ignoring it completely. They can't step up until you're arguing with them or fighting over it. It's not that they're always actively trying to hurt you or the relationship; it's that their brains don't want them to stop. They have to learn how to control this urge and curb it when it's popping up in full force. They have to learn how to work around the urge to defy or ignore you. They need to get trained out of that behavior, working with a therapist or counselor, or through consequences that take away the desire to engage in the negative behavior. The affected partner isn't necessarily behaving badly on purpose, but they are engaging in behaviors that can destroy the foundation of the marriage.

After identifying the source of the conflict, you can now begin to understand how to eliminate them. One of the biggest sources of conflict in a marriage, especially one affected by ADHD, is that one or both partners feel as though they aren't being heard. For example, one spouse might feel as though they've done everything in their power to explain why they're upset, but unless they know they're being heard, they have no confidence the issue will be resolved satisfactorily. As an example, if Bob is upset that Sara repeatedly ignores him when he asks her to text him after she leaves the office, and Sara says she's listened but continues to forget to do so, Bob is going to feel as though his words went in one ear and out the other.

Becoming a better, more active listener is the next step for both of you. Most of us want to be heard, but we may not listen when someone else speaks. Are you an active listener? Active listening is more difficult for people with the disorder, but it's a skill that can be learned like anything else. Active listening means stopping anything else you're doing when someone wants to talk to you. It means putting down the phone, waiting to send a text, or pausing your video game. It means giving your partner eye contact or demonstrating body language that shows you're engaged in the conversation.

While it might feel tough to engage in a lengthy conversation, there are a few ways you can help yourself remain active. Use a fidget toy that helps you stay focused but doesn't distract your partner. Agree to a time limit for the conversation. Discuss the issue for no more than twenty minutes and then agree to pick it up again later if it's still unresolved. By giving yourself a time limit you're both more likely to focus on what's important. You can also work with your ADHD by going into a quiet, non-stimulating environment to have a discussion. Trying to engage someone with the disorder in a serious talk while there's a lot of environmental stimulation in the background will just be counterproductive. You're more likely to feel frustrated than engaged.

Active listening also ensures you foster a sense of safety and trust in each other. This means that you know you won't be treated badly, punished, or humiliated for speaking up. The two of you are comfortable laying it all on the line and working through problems together without fear of repercussions or backlash. If you want to show you're actively listening and that their concerns are treated seriously, make sure you ask good questions. Asking clarifying questions also helps you stay engaged. With a disorder like ADHD, you may struggle to retain the information, so don't be afraid to repeat the information back to your partner. This allows them to correct or verify what you have heard. Being engaged will help you minimize how your disorder interferes when your partner is attempting to communicate with you.

Another reason conflict can arise in your marriage is because your spouse wants you to put more effort in to be an equal partner or often feels like they're in a parent-child relationship with you. They want you to take a more active role in solving the problems that arise, but you inadvertently push the narrative that you don't care because you're not stepping up. Are you taking the initiative to help when without being asked? Are you finding ways to figure problems out on your own, or waiting for your partner to fix things? Are you engaging in active problem solving, or passively waiting for the issue to just go away on its own? Being an adult can feel tough some days. You have responsibilities that you never imagined, and sometimes you just want to get away from it all. The problem comes when you run away from your responsibilities in a relationship. You're now leaving all the problems at your partner's feet, and it's wildly unfair. Feeling overwhelmed doesn't give you a pass to do nothing.

Starting today, you're going to learn how to become a problem solver and you're going to engage in active problem-solving. When you're unsure how to do something, look it up instead of asking your spouse. There are thousands upon thousands of YouTube videos,

195

WikiHow articles, and blog posts that detail exactly how to do a vast number of adult tasks. No one is born knowing how to do everything, they have to learn, and you are more than capable of doing so. When you feel like your spouse is nagging you, find out what the real issue might be. There's always an underlying issue behind a seemingly petty one. For example, if your spouse is constantly nagging you about taking out the trash, there could be an underlying concern for bugs or rodents, they could be worried about how sanitary things are with children around, or they could be stressed about something outside of their control and having the trash taken out every night is something they feel they can control.

Whatever is the underlying issue, help them by making sure they feel secure in coming to you with their problem. The disorder often means that your partner doesn't always feel comfortable coming to you for help. The ironic thing is that people with the disorder are often great problem solvers. They can think outside the box, look at problems from a different perspective and see things others don't. It's important to hone that problem-solving skill for your relationship. It's useful when coming up with ways to tackle problems in the office, but it's just as helpful in tackling issues at home.

Start by being a safe place for your partner to come to with their issues. Being dismissive or critical won't help. Instead, give them space to be heard. Avoid the urge to be defensive or to dismiss their concerns out of hand. You can't resolve conflict if one or both of you are resistant to hearing what is being communicated. Being a good problem-solver means being a good listener. If they come to you with something they see as an issue, be willing to hear them out before speaking. Sometimes we're ready to jump in and explain things or defend ourselves before we've even let our partner finish talking. Instead, ask if they've said everything they wanted before you jump in. It's not only respectful, but it shows that you're listening instead of just waiting to jump in.

196

When you're given the opportunity to speak, now it's time to show you can be a problem-solver. Start by setting aside your feelings and your ego. It doesn't mean ignoring your feelings or putting yourself second to your partner. It means leaving your emotions out of the equation and treating it like a problem to be solved analytically. When you approach the problem critically, you're less likely to feel anxious or upset about the situation. You're an engineer here to fix something that's not working. First, identify whatever the problem is that's giving you both trouble. Then, try to figure out what's causing the issue. Often it's not just a matter of the affected spouse being the instigator but a breakdown in communication or expectations.

Think up several possible ways to solve the problem. Look over the options and think about what might work. If A doesn't work, have B, C, and D as backup plans. Choose the solution you feel will work best for the problem. Think through the possible outcomes for each before choosing the right one. Then, put that chosen plan into place and watch to see if that works. If not, go back to the drawing board. Continually check to make sure that the solution still works over time. If not, try another avenue. If you're still struggling, seek outside help like advice from a friend or family member.

Here is an example of the way that one couple worked on their conflict resolution together:

Hannah and Jamie have been married for just over a year. Jamie has ADHD and was diagnosed young. She started medication for it in elementary school and took it regularly throughout school until college. After that, she decided to go off it for a break, and that's when she met Hannah. Jamie is currently unmedicated but does her best to manage her symptoms with exercise and meditation. Hannah has noticed that lately Jamie has been busy with school and work and hasn't been exercising as much as she used to. She's also been so tired that she goes to bed early every night, skipping her nightly meditation.

Jamie has also been more snappy with her wife. Hannah has tried to make things easier for her wife while she's in school by taking over most of the household duties, only asking her to contribute to a few tasks. Lately, though, Jamie hasn't even been doing those. Instead, she's been coming home and watching YouTube videos after work and procrastinating on homework until the last minute.

Hannah has tried not to complain because she understands that her wife is busy, but she gets to a point where she starts to resent being in charge of the entire household and working 40-plus hours a week. It feels like her wife can't be bothered to help. She doesn't know what to do anymore. Things reach a boiling point when Hannah asks Jamie to pop a frozen pizza in the oven after a long day of work. She comes home, ready to eat, only to find out that not only did Jamie ignore her text, but the kitchen was a huge mess, so even if she wanted to put a pizza in the oven, it would take time to clear away the mess enough to do so. They end up in a fight, yelling at each other, and Jamie leaves the house in a huff.

Hannah and Jamie are in a conflict. Hannah is fed up with her wife and feels as though she's bent over backward to accommodate Jamie's schedule with no consideration in return. She also feels like her wife has been more argumentative and irate lately, making her difficult to live with. When Jamie cools off, they come back and sit down together to talk about things. She lays it out for Jamie, explaining how she feels. Jamie takes the opportunity to listen to what her wife has to say, giving her space to talk about her feelings and vent her frustrations without interrupting. When Hannah is done speaking, Jamie explains that because of her workload, she's been too exhausted to take time for herself and has been taking out her emotions on her wife. She owns up to the problem, understanding that she's been difficult to live with lately.

Hannah also acknowledges that she could have been better at communicating her needs in a way that works with her wife's ADHD. She understands that nagging Jamie and getting angry hasn't solved the problem for either of them. Jamie admits that she wants to fix things, and she realizes that while she used to have time to exercise a lot and meditate, she no longer has that same time, and her ADHD has been getting worse. She pinpoints the problem at the source. The next step she takes is brainstorming with her wife to develop solutions for her problem. She suggests they take walks on the weekends together, thereby spending time together and giving Jamie some exercise. Hannah likes that but points out that Jamie needs more than a few weekend walks. Jamie thinks it over and decides that the best solution to the problem at the moment is for her to go back on medication. She knows that without the time to exercise and meditate, she can't function as well, and since she has so much on her plate, she decides that she'll talk to her doctor.

The two of them looked at the problem objectively. Hannah didn't blame Jamie for the state of their relationship, and Jamie took responsibility for her part in the problem. They were able to get to the heart of the issue together. They could have worked on fixing those small issues together, hoping that things would change, but they realized that there was a bigger issue at play—namely that Jamie was feeling like her entire life was getting out of control. Jamie knew that if she wanted to fix things, it wouldn't be one simple fix either. Medication would help, but they would still need to work through the issues that were cropping up.

They tried medication, and it definitely started making a difference. The issues didn't completely disappear but things were more manageable for Jamie on the day-to-day. They scheduled a check-in within a month of starting medication so that they could honestly talk about how things were going. Hannah was pleased with the improvement but noted that Jamie was still constantly tired at the end of the day. Jamie admitted that working and going to school was tough for her, even with medication. They mutually decided for Jamie to quit her job. Hannah made enough to support them both, and Jamie knew she would make more once she graduated, and her focus on school, for now, was the best for their relationship and Jamie's mental health.

They knew that the issue was bigger than both of them and that it wasn't about who was right or wrong–it was about coming together to look at the problem, pinpoint where the issue was exactly, and brainstorm ways to fix it. Often in high-conflict situations, things aren't as black and white as "My spouse is ignoring me and only focusing on themselves!" Or "My partner won't ever listen to me!" Getting to the heart of the matter is vital. It means that you can eliminate the growth at the root, instead of getting bogged down by smaller, petty issues. If the problem can be eliminated at the source, many of the smaller issues will also be eliminated as well.

Chapter Summary

- Conflict arises when two or more people have different opinions and can't come together on them without work. For example, an affected marriage can have conflict because of the way the symptoms present–difficulty with understanding other's points of view, difficulty with following through, lack of empathy for the other's emotions, and troubles with self-esteem affecting criticism.
- The best way to handle conflict is to become a better listener and a better problem solver. Becoming a better listener requires setting aside your ego and engaging in active listening. Active listening means staying engaged, asking good questions, and using affirmative language to show you sympathize.

- Becoming a better problem solver includes admitting to the problem, looking at the options, figuring out the best ones, trying that out through trial and error, and continually checking in to ensure that the solution still works.

Do you feel like the problem with your conflicts lies with how you communicate? If it's a communication issue causing conflict, the next chapter will discuss communication. You'll learn how to communicate with each other.

Day Five: Improve Communication

Exercise: Do this at the end of each week. Sit in a comfortable position, in an intimate place for the two of you. Bedroom, couch, anywhere you feel comfortable. Face each other. You can hold hands if you wish. Look each other in the eye, breathing in and out deeply until you both feel calmness and stillness inside.

Each of you takes turns listing out the things you were grateful the other did that week. Start with broad things such as "I'm grateful you were by my side every night at bedtime" and work down to more specific examples such as "I'm grateful you made a delicious dinner on Friday." Do this 5 to 10 times. Repeat the exercise each week to build gratitude into your daily life.

Do you feel like you have to repeat yourself for your spouse to understand or comprehend what you're saying? Do you feel your partner often gives you only vague information about their day? Maybe you experience issues with your spouse explaining themselves clearly–especially when they've done something to upset you.

One of the ways that ADHD affects relationships is in the area of communication. Marriages affected by ADHD can have higher instances of miscommunication, especially misunderstandings, hurt feelings, and lack of communication. More than that, there are also ways in which we could be misunderstanding our partner's intentions or even misinterpreting them. It can feel like the disorder hijacks your conversations, leading you to interrupt people, or your lack of attention span causes you to miss important details in conversations.

It's possible to hog the conversation, especially if you feel passionate about the topic, leading others to feel like they have no space to talk.

Whatever it is, you may feel like trying to fix it has your brain working against itself. That's true–and it's because of your executive dysfunction. Executive functions are part of the cognitive processes of your brain–kind of like your brain's manager–that regulate and control certain abilities such as self-control, organization, time management, memory, and emotional regulation. Executive dysfunction is "a term used to describe the range of cognitive, behavioral, and emotional difficulties which occur as a result of [a] disorder or a traumatic brain injury." (Rodden & Saline 2022) People who struggle with executive dysfunction struggle with things like staying on task, planning, staying organized, and the ability to regulate their emotions. They also struggle with self-restraint and self-awareness. These are all difficulties that can add up to much bigger problems in relationships.

As marriage is a give-and-take endeavor, it can feel as though the non-affected partner is doing all the giving while the disordered partner is doing all the taking. When the affected partner is upset, they may lash out instead of calmly expressing themselves. It is a real struggle for the affected partner to regulate their emotions at the moment, and this definitely can lead to hurt feelings. Additionally, the affected partner could be struggling to articulate whatever is affecting or bothering them that contributes to the issues they're experiencing. They also struggle with non-verbal communication, as we discussed on day three. As a result, they don't understand how or why they have upset you or how you're expressing your frustration.

People with the disorder also struggle to process information and tend to internalize issues. They often struggle with comorbidities such as anxiety and depression. They take what you're saying as an attack on them or disappointment in who they are as a person. Their brains want to assign meaning to everything to understand and look for ways to pick apart whatever you communicate. Anxiety and depression also look for ways to turn their thoughts against themselves. It's a cycle perpetuated by past negative experiences.

It's not that they're looking for ways to be hurt; it's that their brains struggle to process. For some, it's about understanding when they're talking too much and not listening enough. For others, it's about finding the words to communicate how they feel. It will take baby steps to improve communication, but it can be done. The best way to go about it is to understand that communication is a two-way street. It's not going to be easy to communicate if the affected partner feels bad about how they communicate. And it's not going to be easy to manage if the affected partner doesn't communicate at all.

As a child, did you ever get a report card that said, "Good student, but they talk too much in class"? Were you labeled a chatterbox growing up? Do you accidentally dominate conversations? Talking too much or in excess is one of the disorder's symptoms. You may not even realize you're doing it. It can be easy for you to go on and on if you're excited about the topic. Talking too much could be driving your spouse up the wall, though. They feel as if they can't get a word in edgewise, or they feel like you're not taking time to listen to them. Do you rush to explain yourself and end up overexplaining? You're probably so eager to fix the situation that you're not letting your partner communicate their needs.

It's okay to be excited or passionate about something. It's okay to want to explain yourself when situations crop up. It's also necessary to let the conversation flow a little more. One way to combat it when you feel like you're talking too much is to ask questions after you've spoken for a few sentences. This lets the other person have a say and gives the conversation a more natural flow. If you repeat the things they say to yourself silently, you can keep focused on listening to your partner instead of talking. When dealing with a discussion or argument, if you feel like you're talking too much, it's okay to pause and ask your partner if they have something to add. This ensures that you both get a fair chance to speak.

Sometimes you do your best not to talk too much, but you end up interrupting anyway. When you interrupt others, it can come across as rude, thoughtless, or bossy. You make others feel like you don't give them enough respect to listen. It can be hard; you get so excited that you want to jump in, or you worry that they'll move the conversation along before you get a chance to add your piece. You also worry that you'll forget what you have to say if you don't say it right then and there. Try to become more aware of how often you're interrupting others when they're speaking. Count the times you interrupt without meaning and work on not interrupting more than a certain amount of times. If you do catch yourself interrupting, take ownership. A simple "I'm sorry for interrupting, what were you going to say?" goes a long way. During conversations, take a deep breath, slowly, and then exhale if you find yourself overwhelmed. You can calm yourself down so the urge to interrupt lessens. With your spouse, give each person a chance to talk without interruption. Cover your mouth with your hands if you need to, or sit on your hands as a reminder not to speak until it's your turn. This works most effectively during a serious discussion, but it can be a good way to practice for less important topics as well.

One reason you are often interrupting is that people with the disorder tend to struggle with short-term memory, and they know if they don't speak as quickly as possible when they have a thought, it will likely be gone before they get a chance to express it. It can certainly be good to quickly express an important thought, but interrupting to do so is considered rude. If you're prone to forgetting, write things down ahead of time, jot a note for yourself on your phone or ask politely to interrupt. Saying "I'm sorry to interrupt, I have a question/I have a thought" can help the other person feel that you're not trying to hog the conversation but understand that you have something to contribute.

If you wait until it's your turn, you also give yourself time to think over what you want to say and decide whether or not it's important to the conversation. Blurting things out that are hurtful, inappropriate, or unhelpful is common with the disorder, and sometimes it's best to take a step back and ruminate over what you want to say.

There's an acronym that can be helpful here. T.H.I.N.K. Ask yourself:

- (T) Is it True?
- (H) Is it Helpful?
- (I) Is it Inspiring?
- (N) Is it Necessary?
- (K) Is it Kind?

Using T.H.I.N.K before you speak can eliminate a lot of hurt feelings, insecurities, and verbal missteps. Try to use the acronym when you're going into a difficult conversation with your spouse. We all get into bad habits of using words that hurt. ADHD amplifies that because you lack the ability to filter unless you work at it. The disorder can make you feel as though you want to lash out, and one of the ways we lash out as humans is to throw exaggerated claims using "always" and "never" which can derail the conversation and put our partner on the defensive. It's very rarely true that someone always or never does something, so try to eliminate that from your vocabulary when you're having a discussion.

On the other hand, you could be struggling to come up with the words to say to express yourself when you're communicating. You feel as though you want your partner to understand you, but the words won't come out, or you use the wrong words, which leads to misunderstandings. When that happens, take a deep breath and work

206

on organizing your thoughts. Ask for a pause so you can collect yourself. If the words still aren't coming to you, ask to talk later. Write down what you want to say and when you reconvene, have your partner read them to you so they can understand what you've said. Ask what they are getting from your words. This will stop any miscommunication in its tracks by cutting it off at the source.

You don't have to resolve every problem straight away. Get in the habit of calling for a time-out when you feel flustered, angry, upset, embarrassed, or anxious and you can't communicate what you want to say right away. By giving yourself time, you are not only letting yourself collect your thoughts, but you give yourself time to calm down as well and deal with the initial feelings that are bombarding you. This is especially relevant during long conversations. ADHD makes it difficult to process and communicate during long discussions. When you find yourself stuck in a long conversation, try to ask for a break or set yourself up for success ahead of time. Eliminate distractions before you talk. Turn off the television, put down the phone, and close the door to avoid interruptions. Ask if you can record the conversation to listen to it again later. This is especially good practice if you're forgetful and you want to remember the important things your partner brought up or important details that you're likely to forget.

Long conversations can be difficult. With ADHD, you zone out, even if you know you want to listen. You know that you're likely to miss important information when you zone out. It's tempting to let yourself zone out. It can even be helpful, to a degree. You're more likely to pay attention if your brain can take "breaks," so to speak. Unfortunately, you end up missing important information or details. Trying to sit through a long conversation without breaks is possible with some of the tools and tips mentioned in the chapter *Day One*, but at some point, you have also to decide if it's worth putting both of yourselves through that stress. Ultimately, working with the disorder is better than working against it. Breaking important conversations up into smaller, more manageable chunks is a lot easier on both partners and a much healthier way of dealing with issues than trying to work through a list of problems over the course of several hours.

Do you, as the non-affected spouse, feel as though you're constantly communicating only to realize that what you said went in one ear and out the other? Do you get angry or anxious that your spouse won't remember what you tell them and nag them so they will remember? Are you using their ADHD against them or working with them? It's easy to blame your spouse for not doing their part, but it's on both of you to communicate better. If you were sick with an illness that meant you were limited in what you could do around the house, would you be upset if your spouse put unfair expectations on you and then got fed up when you couldn't meet those expectations? The disorder is also an illness—it's a mental illness. It means that there are limitations to what your partner can do, and you are putting them to the same unfair standards. In this case, there are no physical limitations, but there are things that you need to work around.

If you desire to have them remember certain important dates, and you know that remembering things is a challenge, help them remember. Set up a household calendar, text them reminders, work with them, and don't expect that they always get it right on their own. If they often interrupt you during conversations, instead of yelling at them or scolding them like a child, gently put your hand on theirs and remind them that it's still your turn. Treat them like an adult but give them the grace that their disorder sometimes needs. Then, when you feel like nagging or berating, take a step back and ask yourself the T.H.I.N.K. questions—is it true, helpful, inspiring, necessary, or kind? Treating each other with more respect will go a long way toward rebuilding the bridge between the two of you, and it can head issues off at the pass.

When you find your spouse struggling to find the right words to say, give them the space they need to speak without interrupting or trying to guess what they might be saying. If their words come out wrong, realize that they don't intend to hurt you, they are struggling to explain the complex way their brain communicates thoughts and emotions to them. Imagine a train going from Los Angeles, CA to Charlotte, NC. On a map, they appear to be almost a straight line across. A journey like that, by train, wouldn't take very long at all in a straight line. However, trains make frequent stops. A journey that looks like two days on a train might be more like ten days with all the stops. The ADHD brain is similar. Thoughts move slower and less linearly for those with the disorder. It takes longer to work from one thought to the next. Being patient with them as they work through their train of thought, no pun intended, will allow them to think through what they want to say. Additionally, ADHD brains are adept at looking at a problem and working through solutions. Giving them time to think will let their brain pick up ideas along the way and arrive at their destination with a fresh solution that neither of you has thought of yet.

The two of you can also work together to find better ways to communicate—ways that work for your unique situation. For example, if you realize that you struggle with verbal communication, you might write each other letters that lay out the words that you can't get out. It gives you both a chance to explain your side without interruption. You should communicate this way only after giving yourself time to calm down. Communication should never be done via text message or email when you're angry, as there is no tone indicator via written communication. If you need to communicate more urgently but still struggle, sit next to each other while you text. This way you have the opportunity to collect your thoughts but can also clarify face to face as well. Another communication hack for affected couples is creating rules for engagement. When you create rules for your discussions or discourse, you are less likely to end up in yelling matches. As an example, create a rule that no name-calling is allowed. If name-calling comes up, agree that the other party calls a time-out immediately, and both parties must walk away.

You could also have a rule that states no use of extreme statements like "always" and "never." If those happen, call for a pause. These statements are often masks for underlying issues, and you want to get to the heart of the issue. It may seem like the frustration is in the instance of the "always" and "never," but there's something deeper going on. When one person uses those extremes, they feel as though their concerns aren't heard. They feel you aren't taking their concerns seriously and don't feel respected. You can also encourage each other to share what you *need* instead of what you *expect*. Emphasizing the facts of what you need instead of putting demands or expectations on them will turn them from feeling defensive into feeling proactive.

Reboot. Sometimes a discussion turns into an argument or a screaming match, and it feels like everything goes wrong in those instances. When the two of you are calming down, give yourselves time to reflect on what went wrong. Often, dealing with the disorder means that you get good at self-reflection in hindsight. You often think of the witty remarks you might have made or better strategies you could have used to diffuse the situation. You also reflect on the mistakes you made that you would do differently if given a chance. Use that to your advantage here. Come back together, and each of you should discuss how *you* would have handled things differently to ensure a positive experience. Extend an olive branch, swallow your pride and admit when you're wrong. There's always opportunities to grow and do better in the future.

Even when we try our best, things still seem to be getting out of control. You can communicate all day long, but nothing will change if the other person won't listen or can't hear what you're saying. Do you feel like you've had all the talks, heard all the promises and nothing is changing? Then, it might be time to seek out professional help. A marriage and family therapist or counselor is trained in handling communication issues and conflict resolution between couples. Seeking out therapy is a good option when the two of you are having more fights than discussions and more arguments than resolutions.

Seeking out help can sometimes feel like admitting defeat. That's not the case, though. We are only human, and in the end, we are limited in our abilities to change without outside help. You get stuck in the mindset that airing your problems is wrong or will somehow magnify them if you admit what's happening. You think that allowing a stranger to know intimate details of your relationship is wrong. You feel like there's no helping the two of you, and going to a therapist won't fix what's broken. These mindsets will hold you back from working through the communication issues preventing you from having a happy, successful relationship. Bringing up the issues in couples counseling can certainly be difficult. But marriage does take work, and good relationships are ones where both partners are ready to do the work.

If you find yourself at a crossroads, especially if you're contemplating divorce, you feel as though there are only two options in front of you. Do you stay, knowing you're unhappy, or do you leave to find happiness elsewhere? You feel stuck and afraid of making the wrong choice. You know it's time to seek help when the issues are bad enough that you're contemplating leaving, but here are some of the other signs it's time to seek help:

- Conflicts have begun to escalate and nasty words are hurled around.

- There is a bridge of emotional distance between you that you can't cross.
- You feel as though you are losing trust in your partner.
- Your partner's own self-worth and fears of abandonment are interfering with your ability to properly communicate without escalation and accusations.
- Your difficulties with in-laws, work stress, or friends are bleeding into your ability to be open and honest with each other.
- You two can't come together to agree on fundamental issues such as parenting styles.
- You feel unsupported or have difficulty opening up to each other emotionally.
- You worry that your partner's addictions (alcohol, drugs, porn, or shopping habits) are getting out of control.
- One or both of you experienced a difficult or traumatic upbringing that has emotionally wounded you and made conflict a bigger deal when it arises.
- Undiagnosed depression or anxiety is making it hard for one partner to function.
- Your ADHD is becoming unmanageable to the detriment of your life and relationship.

If one or more of these issues are causing a rift and making you unhappy enough to consider leaving, a good therapist can work with you to help you through these and potentially save your relationship. You will be able to shine a light on the underlying issues and access feelings that were buried or ignored. Even if your marriage isn't on the rocks, counseling can be a huge positive for the relationship. An ounce of prevention is better than a pound of cure, as the saying goes. You want to stop problems in their tracks before they become bigger and more unmanageable–before they can start to crack the foundation of your relationship. You'll learn how to develop healthy relationship skills, solve communication issues, and learn how to communicate better. Like getting your oil changed every 3,000 miles, going to a "couples check-up" in therapy is good for the health of the relationship. You can get an assessment of how your relationship is doing and work through any minor issues or solve small communication problems with help.

The two of you also get the opportunity to set goals for the relationship. You can set a goal that you work towards, and once you feel confident that goal is met, you can discontinue therapy or just go for regular check-ins every so often. Therapy provides a safe space for the two of you to discuss things that you are having difficulty addressing on your own–everything from communication disconnect to differing on values and even intimacy issues. For example, if you're having communication issues, you may still be stumbling because there's a difference between communication and effective communication. This is especially relevant when major life changes are on the horizon, such as deciding to go back to school, having a baby, taking a new job opportunity, or moving house. These types of transitions can destabilize couples due to the stress and pressure that comes from making decisions and planning things out.

Therapy can offer a great deal of help in many areas but finding the right therapist is essential. You need to do your research together before finding a therapist. Look up the things that they focus on and determine if those align with you as a couple. Some counselors offer religious-based help and some offer help for couples in all areas, including sex therapy. Finding the right therapist is a bit like dating, though. You won't know they're right for you until you sit down with them and meet them. It's okay to decide after the first visit, or the first couple of visits, that the therapist isn't a good fit. You may need to try a few out before finding one you connect with. Pay attention to their

213

approach to your issues. You want to ensure their communication style and the rationale behind their questions makes sense to you. If you're not comfortable opening up to them, you won't do the work they ask. Any homework they assign should explained and make sense.

Once you've found a therapist that you both like, encourage each other to continue seeing the therapist both alone and together until you feel you're reaching your communication goals and you both feel as though you've made sufficient progress on your issues. Continuing individual therapy might also be helpful, even beyond reaching your couple's goals. You get the chance to work through issues that compromise your communication with someone qualified to help. Leaning on your spouse for support is always helpful, but some issues are bigger than they can deal with.

Communication can be difficult in any relationship, but ADHD can easily compound the issues. Their symptoms can leave you feeling disengaged, and your frustration can lead them to feel like a burden. By evaluating how you communicate as a couple, you can discover where communication breakdowns happen. Pay attention to how your spouse receives information. Is it better to write down any requests or errands? Do they focus better when they can have multiple shorter conversations instead of one long one? Ultimately, your marriage and its issues will be completely unique to your situation, so it's important to recognize that your way of solving issues reflects that. When you find what works for you, keep doing that. Check in frequently to ensure that the solution is still working, but stick with it if it is. You will both be much happier and feel more attentive and loving when you find what works.

Chapter Summary

- When communication issues happen in an affected marriage, it can often be due to a disconnect in the way the partners communicate. Symptoms such as short attention spans, trouble with memory and concentration, trouble focusing, and difficulty expressing oneself can lead to both feeling frustrated, angry, and hurt. Discussions lead to arguments which lead to fights, and in the end, no one is happy.

- Some of the most common problems that pop up can be solved by creating rules for engagement–rules that you both stick to when discussing problems. A few examples include eliminating exaggerated statements such as "always" and "never," setting a time limit for the discussion, no name-calling, and making sure you communicate face-to-face, even if you have to use electronic communication.

- When all else fails, it might be time to seek out therapy. Therapy can help you both find ways to open up, manage your underlying issues, and shine a light on the deeper problems in the relationship. Finding the right therapist will help both of you long after you've met your goals as a couple.

In the next chapter, we will talk about common insecurities that crop up in ADHD-affected relationships and how to eliminate those insecurities. We will look at how the disorder can affect self-esteem and self-worth and how to improve those so that feedback feels constructive to both parties.

Day Six: Eliminate Insecurities

Exercise: Find a comfortable position for both of you. Lay down on the bed together, or on a blanket. Breathe in through your nose and out through the mouth. Close your eyes and feel the weight of your body pressing down on you. Move your focus above your head and visualize a stream of warm sunlight flowing down into your bodies and washing away any tension. Imagine it filling up your bodies, from your head all the way down to your toes. The sunlight fills you with a sense of ease.

Imagine the stream traveling slowly up your legs again, into your waist, and then up into your torso. Feel it move through your chest, spreading to your shoulders and back and down into your arms, into your hands and fingers. Let any last areas of tension go as it moves up into your neck and throat. Imagine it moving into your face and up into the very top of your head. Allow yourself to simply sit inside the feelings of warmth, comfort, and calming.

Let go of the image in your own time and open your eyes. Recognize how you felt in that moment and create an intention to carry the awareness into the rest of the day.

In a perfect world, no one would suffer from low self-esteem or poor self-image. Unfortunately, many people in the world do, and this can disproportionately affect those with the disorder. Rates of depression, anxiety, additional disorders such as Oppositional Defiant Disorder (ODD), Obsessive-Compulsive Disorder (OCD), and addictive behaviors appear higher than those with ADHD. They are more prone to serious comorbidities, they also experience higher rates of bullying, ostracization, and difficulty making and keeping friends. These are all tied up together and in the bigger picture, mean that those with the disorder are more likely to internalize conflict and struggle

216

with criticism. This can lead to them checking out of the marriage, too stressed that they don't measure up to some ideal, and deciding not to try instead of constantly feeling as though they are a disappointment.

Additionally, the non-affected spouse feels ignored during conversations and lonely when their partner's hyperfocus pulls them away for long periods of time. You feel as though you constantly have to manage your partner's feelings and avoid things that may cause them to explode. You feel rejected when they make insensitive comments or deeply hurt when they hurl insults specifically designed to target your areas of weakness. You feel as though you are the only dependable one, the only one who can get things done. You start to resent your spouse and feel insecure about the state of your relationship. Finances have you feeling as though you're constantly on the verge of being broke because of your partner's spending habits. You look at your spouse and wonder if they really love you. Do they even care? Are you in this marriage alone? You wonder if they can fall out of love as easily as they seemed to fall in love with you.

"[People with] ADHD labor more than others to define who we are and figure out where we fit. Our brains work faster and that can be exhausting or frustrating. Everyone else has to catch up." (Steed, 2022) You may work extra hard to make people like you, leading you to talk over others, interrupt, or dominate social situations. You relate to other people by sharing your own stories and trying to be the life of the party. You want to be liked, so you come across as charismatic or flirty. When you work so hard to be the center of attention, you come across as self-centered and self-absorbed. Your partner may feel you're not really engaged in the conversation; you're just waiting for a break to one-up their story or get a laugh. They feel you don't really care about what they have to say. Your partner feels like the joy is being sucked from the relationship and their insecurities may get the better of them. You struggle to understand why your partner has doubts about the relationship. The two of you aren't on the same page, and things are deteriorating. What can you do when this happens?

The ADHD brain can often be self-sabotaging, leading to contradictory behavior that doesn't make sense, even to the affected partner. When you don't understand your own brain, you can't communicate what you're thinking or feeling to your partner. Unfortunately, your brain likes to only pick up on criticism. You hear your partner say, "You don't listen to me" and "I'm having doubts about whether or not I really love you." Your instinct is to defend yourself instead of listening to what they're saying to you. This can cause a breakdown in communication. You want to protect yourself from what you see as criticism, so you're ready to lash out and turn the tables.

It also burrows into your brain. You end up hyperfocused on the negatives. When your hyperfocus kicks into overdrive, you end up replaying the negative messages in your brain repeatedly, obsessing about them. You analyze every word and every action to see where you went wrong and how you can fix it. This can kick up your anxiety and depression. You become overwhelmed or numb. Your brain exaggerates the issues or conjures up imagined scenarios. As your brain tries to analyze and fix what's happening, and as you obsess over it more and more, you create your own reality that stands in stark contrast to the truth. Even small things become big problems inside your head. You try to numb the pain by engaging in escapist behavior– whether that's sitting alone playing on your phone for hours, drinking, or making major decisions–such as leaving the country.

You also end up overthinking yourself to the point of destruction. You quit your job because you feel like you're never going to be good enough. You move far away to get a fresh start–only to realize that you desperately miss home. Or, you break up with your partner because you think they deserve better, or that you need to fix yourself before you can be with them. You don't want to get into this mindset because it's self-defeatist thinking. By breaking up or quitting your job, you fulfill the idea that you're not good enough instead of taking responsibility for your mistakes and working towards the clean slate you really want—in the job or relationship. Your problems won't go away if you run away. You're just in a new place with the same problems. Lack of self-love is the root cause of most insecurities. With the way your brain works, you can be your own worst enemy in relationships. You have to learn how to hack your brain and become your own wingman instead.

You don't want to end up in a situation where your insecurities get the better of you. When we let our insecurities drive us, we can end up in situations that crack the foundation of the relationship. Don't let yourself go unchecked with your insecurities. It can push your partner away or tempt you into making terrible decisions that you can never recover from, such as infidelity, crippling debt, addiction issues, or becoming controlling and abusive towards you your partner. This applies to both spouses equally, as the non-affected partner can let their insecurities easily overwhelm them as well. Learn to recognize the signs of insecurity in yourself before they become too much to handle. For example, recognize when you're becoming jealous, angry, self-centered, or argumentative. Your fear will lead to anger, which can lead to hatred, ending with both of you suffering the consequences.

So how do you build confidence in your relationship again? You have to start by building your own self-esteem. There are many ways your brain will try to tell you that you're a bad person, too messed up for love, or that you're not worthy of happiness. Working through those feelings won't be easy. You will always encounter failures in your life. Your mistakes don't define you, though. It's the way you act afterward that counts. Regaining your self-esteem as an adult takes work but will make you feel more secure in yourself, your life, and your purpose. "The core beliefs that shape self-esteem are determined by whether a person appreciates and likes who they are." (Jaksa, 2021) You have to work through the negative self-talk, doubts, and obsessive thoughts before you can get to the place you want to be mentally, where you finally like yourself.

You get into the habit of equating your own mistakes as part of your self-worth while dismissing others' mistakes as simply a mistake. You need to focus on recognizing when negative thoughts appear, challenge those thoughts, and dismiss them. Some people equate their inner voice to someone they don't like or a fictional villain. For example, the unpleasant Professor Dolores Umbridge from *Harry Potter*. They assign a personality to the voice, and it becomes easier to imagine it coming from that person. Professor Umbridge is speaking up, saying "You're worthless, you can't do anything right," and then they can roll their eyes at Umbridge, who is evil and obviously trying to upset them. They take control of their thoughts by understanding that reality is what you make of it. Their thoughts have less power over them. These messages are a kind of cognitive distortion. Your brain wants to view things a certain way to filter out anything that doesn't fit in with that message and dismiss evidence to the contrary.

Another way to stop those negative thoughts in their tracks is to understand and accept your diagnosis. The more you understand what's going on, the more you realize that your negative thoughts are coming from your ADHD. You know that your brain struggles with time management, for example, so if you find yourself running late to important events, instead of beating yourself up, accept that your brain just works differently than others, and you have to manage it differently. It is not a disease; it's a disorder of the brain. It's nothing to be ashamed of or embarrassed by, and you should learn to love who you are, all of you, the ADHD parts included. You should also make an effort to stop comparing yourself to other people. When you compare their best with your worst, you're going to come out looking bad, but it's an inherently flawed train of logic. People only show their highlight reels, the best parts of their lives. You have no idea what goes on behind the scenes in other people's lives.

Instead of focusing on your failures or disappointments, work on identifying and appreciating your accomplishments. Take stock of the things you're proudest of and recognize what that means in the grander scheme. Have you done something unique? Have you gotten an education? Have you created something? Do you have children in your life? You have things about you that are special and worth celebrating. If journaling is something you enjoy, start a gratitude journal that focuses on the things in your life that you're proud of and things that you've accomplished, big or small. Review your journal at the end of every week to see how you've grown and changed. You may be surprised at how much this boosts your self-esteem. You're training your brain to focus on the good instead of filtering it out. Change is easier to see when you can track it.

If you feel like you have a lot of areas where you want to grow, sit down and assess your strengths and weaknesses. Make a list of what you're good at and what you want to improve on. If you want to improve, you have to set realistic and attainable goals. Set goals for the short-term, the medium, and the long-term. Set goals for three months, six months, and one year. Break down your goals into manageable chunks. Then, check in with yourself to make sure that the goals are still attainable and don't beat yourself up if you're not meeting them. It doesn't mean you're a failure; it just means you need to reevaluate your time frame. When you give yourself grace, you may find that you accomplish a lot more than you ever thought you could.

When problems arise in your life, focus on being a problem-solver. You can easily get paralyzed by indecision or feel like you don't know what to do. The secret is, most people don't really know what they're doing–they just get great at winging it. Take charge when you see a problem and ask yourself, "What can I do about it?" Be proactive, and if worst comes to worst, fake it till you make it. If you mess up, oh well, at least you tried. Trying is much better than doing nothing, and you learn something about handling the situation in the future. Don't "should" yourself. Get past the "I could/should/would have done" and tell yourself "I will" and "I can" instead. Putting yourself out there is scary, but you won't know if you can until you attempt to do it. You will also learn more about yourself in the process. It's never too late to learn how to manage and grow with ADHD.

When you're trying to gain self-confidence, you have to ensure you're surrounding yourself with positive people as well. Negative people or relationships will bring you down and make you feel insecure or bad about yourself. You may not notice it right away, but think about the times you've been around people who are constantly complaining to you. You start to complain a lot too, don't you? Or you start to feel angry and upset on their behalf, and then your own life seems unsettled. People who have poor attitudes will bring you down with them. Misery loves company, so to speak. When you are surrounded by positive people, you start to feel better about yourself, your life, and your place in the universe. You can embrace the good and understand that the bad isn't all that bad. By pushing yourself to move away from negative relationships and adopt ones with positive people, you will notice a change in your self-esteem and self-confidence.

Are you being kind to yourself when you make a mistake? Sometimes we want to blame our ADHD or despair that we will never be able to make good decisions because of it. Your disorder can be a challenge for you, but it's not all you are. We often feel as though everyone is judging us for our mistakes or dwelling on the words we spoke, but the reality is, people don't usually remember things like that. You might remember an embarrassing moment at work or cringe when you recall something you said to a friend, but they have likely already forgotten it. You should be kinder to yourself and remind yourself that those little moments will pass from their minds without further thought. You don't need to beat yourself up over it, especially if you own up and take responsibility right away. You forgive other people for minor errors or faults; practice forgiving yourself as well. Being able to forgive yourself will go a long way towards building your confidence back up. You are more than the sum of your mistakes, and you should push yourself to recognize that.

Try to avoid criticizing yourself too harshly in front of others as well. Not only can it reinforce your own negative view of yourself, but it can also make others view you with lower expectations or opinions unfairly. People are most attracted to those with self-confidence. Those who are self-assured are interesting. They present themselves as someone worth knowing. It's tiring to be around someone who always puts themselves down. It's draining. You unintentionally push people away by putting yourself down in front of others. You put out there what you will get back. If you're constantly critiquing yourself and putting yourself down, those attracted to you will draw in people who are just as negative and draining. If you focus on the good things about yourself and bring self-confidence to the table, you'll be able to attract positive people who will, in turn, bring you up as well.

Take small steps forward when you work on your self-image and self-esteem. Of course, you will stumble and make mistakes, and it's tempting to berate yourself, but you need to acknowledge that it's part of the journey; it's part of the learning and growing that you're doing. Track your progress with your therapist or with a journal. Look back every so often to see how you've grown. It might not be obvious in a week, but looking once a month can show you how far you've come. Celebrate your small victories, and revel in your tiny accomplishments. Whatever you need to do to push yourself to recognize the good inside of you. You want to focus on that, not the things that trip you up or make you doubt yourself.

Having positive self-esteem is all about asking yourself two questions: "So what?" and "What's next?" You'll do stupid things, make dumb mistakes, act inappropriately, offend people, or make a fool out of yourself throughout your lifetime. When that happens, you have to stop and ask yourself, So what? What is the big deal? What is the problem? So you accidentally spilled coffee on yourself. So you forgot to turn an assignment in for class? What is the worst that can happen? Seriously, think of the worst things that might happen to you as a result. Let yourself think through the ridiculous scenarios in your head and then ask yourself, "What's next?" How will you deal? How will you fix your mistakes? How will you prevent it so that those dire consequences don't happen? Taking the time to imagine the worst-case can often make you feel better, recognize when you're being silly and when you need to take the proper responsibility. Learning how to separate your silly moments from true moments of growth will help you recognize that there's way more good in you than bad, more positive than negative, and more to like than dislike.

When it comes to working on your self-esteem, your partner should be your ally in this. It's time to examine how you're talking to each other and how you provide feedback. Are you inadvertently tearing each other down? You might be surprised that your actions have an effect on your spouse and on your marriage. Learning how to communicate needs is important but so is learning how to give good feedback. When it comes to providing feedback, are you doing so to encourage your spouse to come to you when they make a mistake or are you making them fear your reaction? Are the two of you able to effectively communicate your needs, or do you place demands on your partner? They should be able to approach you with any problem and feel confident that you will be a safe place for them. If you feel like you're both struggling to be that person, you are contributing to each other's insecurities without realizing it. As a result, you are both unintentionally pushing each other away emotionally.

So how do you start changing things around? You have a new skill to learn–how to be a positive source of feedback for each other. Start by making sure that both of you are actually safe places for the other person to come to. When something goes wrong, make sure that your partner can trust that if they come to you with the problem, you aren't going to berate, belittle, humiliate, or hold it against them at a later point. When you're dealing with a disorder like ADHD, mistakes *will* happen. To ensure that your partner doesn't lie to you or hide their mistakes, you want to be a person that makes them feel that it's okay to make a mistake. Without trust, relationships have no foundation to grow. Establishing that trust is key to ensuring that your partner knows they can talk to you about it if something goes wrong. You also want to ensure that you ask if the issue is one that they need help fixing or if they just want to vent about it. When you push to fix the problem, they might feel resentful or that you don't trust them to fix their own error.

It's also important that you provide a balanced perspective if you have to give your partner feedback. Sometimes it's necessary for the relationship to talk about what is and what isn't working. The ADHD brain wants to take critique as criticism immediately, and it's important to know how to do that. Balancing the positive with the negative is part of that. Let them know the things you see that are good–any growth or positive changes–before diving into whatever issues you might be having. Learning how to balance your perspective is a good way to ensure that your spouse knows you still care, that their mistakes aren't making you lose love for them, and that you're both able to be on the same page through the discussion. Try to ensure that you're not being overly critical either. When you don't know where to draw the line, you can push your partner to the point of anxiety or frustration. They may feel as though they don't know how to make you happy and push you away or no longer make an effort.

When you need to give feedback, make sure you're giving observations and not interpretations. The fastest way to start an argument is to assign meaning to whatever your partner is doing that is bothering you. Instead, pull them to the side and state the observations that you've come across. For example, say "I've noticed that you haven't been telling me about work lately" instead of "You haven't been talking about work lately, I think you're hiding something." The difference is that one is simply an observation, the other is an accusation. Focus on what you need instead of what they're doing wrong. You want them to rise to meet your needs instead of giving up and feeling that nothing they do is right.

Think about how you're going to respond to their reaction. You can control the way you communicate with them, but you can't control how they react to you. Imagine that they get upset; how are you going to respond? If you react with the same level of emotion, you're liable to take a discussion and turn it into an argument or a fight. What you want to do instead is to anticipate how they react and prepare for them. If they get hostile, angry, or defensive, you need to remain calm without being condescending or without infantilizing them. Avoid attacking their character when you're trying to give feedback as well. It's all too easy to fall into the habit of throwing out personal attacks when you're trying to discuss an issue, but the more you do this, the more you're tearing down the person you're supposed to love. Those with the disorder are likely to take personal attacks to heart even more than those unaffected. It can feel like your world is crashing down around you when you hear your partner tell you what you've already been berating yourself about in your head. It gives weight to the harsh words that you already say to yourself.

Your partner might not appreciate what you have to say, so you need to be prepared for them to be unwilling to meet all your expectations. Be willing and ready to compromise. What's the most important thing for you in this issue? How can you adequately achieve that without giving up on your needs? You may have to give up part of your desires to satisfy your partner's own needs. Be prepared to admit when you're wrong too. Sometimes we go into a discussion with all the fire inside, ready to launch a missile at our partner for doing something we don't like or see as wrong. It's entirely possible to be misreading a situation or misunderstanding where your partner is coming from, and this is when you need to serve yourself a slice of humble pie, swallow your pride and admit you were wrong. Your partner will respect you more for admitting that you're wrong.

On the other hand, sometimes, no one is wrong. Sometimes, it's about accepting that your partner is just that way and there's no right or wrong person. For example, if you're constantly upset about your partner leaving their dirty clothes on the floor, you can spend your marriage miserable and berating them for doing it, or you can accept that it's just a part of who they are and that if they haven't changed yet, they aren't likely to change. Letting that go might feel like you're losing at first, but the ultimate win is learning how to make your marriage work. Choosing to accept them doesn't mean defeat. It means that you love them despite their flaws and that you have chosen to pick your battles. This can help your partner feel less insecure because they know that they are loved and that you're both choosing not to sweat the small stuff.

Learning to be more assertive can also help the two of you eliminate those insecurities. Your partner doesn't have to guess when you're open about what you want and how you want it. You can't expect your partner to be a mind-reader. Sometimes we complain that our partners aren't doing things for us, such as making a big deal of our birthdays or buying flowers for us each week, but are we actually communicating that need with them or just expecting that they do it "because?" When it feels like your partner isn't doing what you want, you need to speak up and make sure that you're communicating your needs to them. If you want flowers every week, ask for it. It probably feels as though the spontaneity and romance are lessened by asking, but isn't it better to ask and get what you want than to complain that your partner isn't doing something they have no idea they should be doing?

Similarly to learning how to be more assertive, it's important to learn when and how to say no to your partner. If you frequently take on more of a load than you can handle, and then you find yourself angry at your partner for their insensitivity, the blame falls on you if you haven't mastered the ability to say "no." In an affected marriage, it can be easy to feel as though you *have* to be there for your spouse no matter what, because they can't do it all by themselves. That's both infantilizing and self-sacrificial. You're in a relationship of equals, and you have to learn that saying no can not only ease your burden but empower your spouse as well. They may get complacent with having you do all the things they can't. They may stop trying or growing if they think you'll handle the things they forget about or mess up. The best way to save the relationship from becoming one that is more parent-child is to learn how to say no. Your spouse still needs you in some ways but not in all ways. The two of you just need to decide what is a vital part of helping them cope with their disorder and what is enabling them to learn and growing on their own.

At the end of the day, the two of you are partners, but you need to open up about the things keeping you from becoming closer and making you feel more secure in the relationship. When you share those parts of yourself, you may be surprised at how much the relationship grows and blossoms.

Chapter Summary

- Insecurities in affected relationships are a common result of the disorder's symptoms–both for the affected partner and the non-affected partner. People with the disorder have difficulty navigating social situations, poor understanding of social cues, lack of empathy for others, and take things personally. This can lead to both partners feeling insecure when their needs aren't met.
- Improving self-esteem is one of the best ways to address the insecurities that build up for those with ADHD. Learning how to love yourself, take care of yourself, and see your own self-worth is important to the relationship's health.
- Both of you need to work on how you handle giving and receiving feedback in the relationship. Giving constructive criticism in a way that nurtures a positive relationship is just as important as learning how to accept critique.

In the next chapter, we will go over how to foster more love and empathy in your relationship, and how to grow as a couple.

Day Seven: Foster empathy and love

Exercise: Get a pen and paper before you sit down. Sit together in a comfortable place. Do this exercise once every six months or as often as needed. Close your eyes and breathe for a moment until you're both relaxed.

Write down ten ways your partner shows you their love. Share your lists out loud. Next, write down ten more ways your partner has grown in the last six months, then share again. Finally, write down ten things you both want to see in your relationship within the next six months.

When stuck in a cycle of issues with an affected partner, it can feel like there's no getting out. There was a reason the two of you fell in love in the first place. And there is a reason that the two of you have made it work as long as you have. If you two are committed to making it work, you need to get yourself out of your roles. It's way too easy to feel that you, as the non-affected partner, have to step into a parental role to help your spouse. It's easy to feel you'll never get it right, so why bother trying as the affected spouse. If you unintentionally get stuck in those roles, your marriage will suffer. You need to learn how to break free of those roles and find a new normal. It's the only way that the both of you will be able to help grow and nurture the relationship going forward.

Fostering a positive, loving relationship isn't hard, but it might take work, depending on where you two are in the relationship at the moment. If you're feeling distant, it will be harder to get back to where you were before. Mutual trust, respect, and love are the foundations for a healthy relationship. It's a choice that you make each day–a choice to get up and make your partner a priority each and every day. In an affected relationship, it may take extra work on the part of both partners. Affected relationships mean making extra choices and doing extra work for the relationship's health. It can feel like its difficult to muster empathy when you've told your spouse to take the dog out and they have forgotten for the hundredth time. Or when you're struggling to like *yourself* and your spouse is mad because you haven't shown them enough affection.

Empathy is all about putting yourself in each other's shoes and letting yourself see yourself from your partner's perspective. Take an evening and walk each other through a day in the life, being detailed and explaining what tasks you do and how those make you feel. Take turns sharing without interruption. You'll be surprised at what you don't think about that your partner does or the things that you take for granted that your partner works to accomplish. It will open your eyes to the things that the two of you do for each other. When learning how to see life from the other's perspective, it's necessary to understand what you go through day-to-day to understand how you might be adding to the other's emotional burden without realizing it. You want to do this in a way that doesn't promote hostility or anger. This is an exercise all about looking through the other's eyes for a moment.

When working toward fostering a new relationship of love and empathy, you want to encourage change to happen as well. After learning about the other's perspective, commit that you're both going to work on reducing any of the other person's burdens you could inadvertently be causing. Start by asking your partner what you can do during the day, every day, to make them feel cared for and loved. These can be as simple as a request to hold hands while walking together or as helpful as requesting that you take on one chore they hate. Whatever you pick, make sure it's something that they can do reasonably well and doesn't add to their burden in other ways. By making these gestures intentional, you are showing how much you care. It isn't about the gesture itself but the intent behind it. Keep in mind the emotional labor that goes into your gestures. It's nice to be brought fresh flowers, but you add to their labor if you expect that they are the ones who have to cut them down and put them in a vase. Make the gesture thoughtful in a proactive way. If they have to work to enjoy the gift, it's not really a gift.

One simple way to add meaningful empathy and love back into your relationship is to take time out of your schedules to incorporate deeper discussions. Often, we get bogged down by the mundane, day-to-day, and we don't have time for those kinds of discussions. Those affected by the disorder love to share their wealth of knowledge on the topics they're passionate about, and the two of you can really learn from each other when you talk about goals, desires, dreams, interests and even your fears. Find out if their dreams have changed or if they have new dreams. Learn about their desires for the future, what they are currently most interested in, and what they've been learning about. Ensure that your attention is solely focused on the other person when you are having these discussions. They will feel important to you, loved by you, and appreciated when you give them your full attention at such an intimate moment.

The way you respond to them in conversation matters as well. You want to respond to tough things with sympathy and not make it about you, which can be difficult for those with the disorder, as that's how they relate to the world. Instead of saying, "I know how you feel, I went through something just like that," try responding, "That sounds terrible. I went through something similar and felt horrible. How do you feel about it?" You're building empathy for the other person and making it a safe space to share their feelings. You also want to learn to laugh together, at your mistakes, at each other's silly misunderstandings, and occasionally, at the absurdity of life. You have to learn to laugh when things are going wrong, as it's a good way to cope instead of giving in to the feelings of despair and anxiety that can overwhelm you. ADHD can cause you to do some pretty silly or weird things if you think about it. Learning to laugh at your disorder will also help you cope better when it seems to be taking everything to manage it.

When trying to grow the love in your relationship, it's also important to be able to forgive and forget. You will both make mistakes. You will both do things that unintentionally hurt the other person. Holding grudges, holding their past mistakes over their heads, and refusing to forgive will damage the relationship. Being able to forgive can seem easy. You may think you struggle more with being able to forget, but sometimes we say we forgive our partner on the surface even if we haven't really done so deep down. Letting go of the past means letting go. It means not bringing it up again. It means truly being able to move on from whatever your partner did. If you can't do that, you won't have a relationship anymore. It's easy to acknowledge and forgive our own shortcomings as the non-affected partner. We need to extend that same grace to our spouse. You want to treat them the way you want to be treated, which means learning to let go of the hurt. It doesn't have to happen right away, but it's an essential step in learning to grow the love and empathy in your relationship.

Be committed to each other and to your commitment too. ADHD can mean that you're craving new, exciting, and different experiences, and that can lead to destructive behaviors like wandering eyes or, at the worst, cheating. Similarly, as the affected spouse, you may find yourself seeking emotional comfort from another when problems get too hard to handle with your spouse. This is when you need to cling to each other the hardest. You have to be committed harder to the idea of the relationship than you are tempted to stray to reel yourself back. The grass is greenest where you water it, after all.

So how do you get back that spark, that feeling you had when you first met? How do you fall in love with your partner all over again? Experts agree that barring abuse or criminal acts, you can always find your way back into the arms of your partner and fall in love with them again.

Falling in love the first time seemed easy, didn't it? It can be that easy again. You just have to do a little bit of work. Are the two of you actively engaging in time together, apart from responsibilities and children, at least once a month? You need to continue to date each other. Dating is how the two of you connected in the first place. Rekindle the spark with a weekly or bi-monthly date night. You both deserve a break, and you deserve to spend time together. Whether taking a walk together, getting dinner outside the house, or spending a whole weekend away–make each other a priority and make time for each other again. You are supposed to be each other's best friends and it's important that you act like each other's best friends. Build each other up, share important things that happen to you–and be willing to listen–to connect. Connection is a vital part of your marriage. According to research, couples who focus on maintaining their friendship are more likely to be able to move past issues and repair the relationship successfully. When the two of you come up against an obstacle together, treat your partner how you would treat your best friend instead of placing blame or treating your spouse like an infant.

Just as it's good to spend time together, make sure you're also spending time apart. Those with ADHD often need a lot of downtime to recharge and recollect themselves. Even if you're not affected by the disorder, it's still good to have time for yourself and by yourself. It may seem counterintuitive to the relationship–when you're trying to fix what's broken–to spend time apart, but absence does indeed make the heart grow fonder. We find ourselves able to regroup and renew our minds and spirits when we're alone, and it gives us time to miss our spouses as well. We start to see our partners in a more positive light and remember the good in them that we fell in love with in the first place. We have the energy to devote to the relationship when we can rest and recharge. We can deal with issues or problems that arise, give our spouses the attention they deserve, and remind ourselves what it's all about.

You should, of course, have your own hobbies and interests. All healthy individuals should have their own interests outside the mundane and outside of the relationship. Cultivating your own interests is vital for your mental health. However, it's important to do things together as a couple Find a hobby, activity, or sport that the two of you might enjoy together–such as surfing or hiking, taking a pottery or dance class together, or having your own mini book club. Spend time on that hobby together each week too. Read your books, work out or practice to improve. Build each other up too. Sometimes we get down on ourselves about our abilities, especially if we see our spouse doing "better" and may feel discouraged about continuing. Make sure that the two of you are on a team together, not trying to compete. Nothing kills the romance faster than when one spouse makes it into a competition. There is a time and a place for friendly competition but this is about the two of you coming together to spend time together. Additionally, make sure you're going out and trying new things together, too. The ADHD brain craves new, different, and exciting things to keep its dopamine supply going. They want to feel the serotonin flooding their brains. So keep it fed and happy by experiencing new and fun things together. Try adventurous activities like skydiving or more subdued ones like exploring the culinary fare your city offers.

Spontaneity is another good way to keep an ADHD brain engaged. Sometimes we get bogged down by the every day, the mundane, and the day-to-day, and we don't put enough room in the schedule for spontaneous trips to the beach or going camping for the weekend on a moment's notice. It's healthy and good to have a little spontaneity in your lives. It can be simple as well. Getting their favorite candy bar or treat for them when you go to the grocery store or sticking a sweet note in their lunch can go a long way. Romance is all about showing the other person that they care. Love languages are a great way to explore how the other gives and receives their love. Remember to take your results with a grain of salt–but there is still truth to be found in it. Sometimes we receive love differently than we show our love, and it can help to understand your partner's perspective on your kind gestures. It's not that they're ungrateful, but mowing the lawn once a week might not feel as loving to them as spending quality time together or being cuddled in bed at night.

Don't forget to speak like you want to be spoken to. It always feels good to be complimented or praised for something, especially if the one giving it notices a change that you've been working on. Practice what you want by giving your partner those compliments, engaging in meaningful praise that shows you notice and appreciate the changes they've made or how they have grown since you first fell in love. Affirm your relationship by pointing out what you love about your spouse and what you love about the two of you as a couple. Whether that's complimenting how hard they've worked on getting that promotion or affirming how much you love living your best lives with your three cats, it reaffirms that you made the right choices.

There are a lot of ways that couples can reconnect when it comes to intimacy. If you feel as though you're lacking in the bedroom, start with ensuring that your partner's needs are met. For men, they need to feel desired and appreciated. For women, they need to feel valued and emotionally connected. If you're struggling to meet their needs, they may not feel reciprocal desires. It's also important to build intimacy slowly. In order to get that spark back, you need to find what lit the flame to begin with. Then, focus on recreating that initial desire. Fan the flames by moving from there to casual physical intimacy. Light touches, reaching for their hand in public, kisses on the cheek, etc. It's best to keep the contact at the level your partner is comfortable with. Some women find it hard to be physically intimate after the birth of a child, for instance, and often find that their partner trying to initiate contact through random groping can make them feel less desired and less likely to want intimacy. Try asking if you can give them a gentle, slow massage instead. Don't expect it to lead anywhere; you're still building intimacy. Put the work in if you want the results.

When it comes to ADHD, you both might think that having the disorder means learning to live with it, and accept that it comes with plenty to make you annoyed or frustrated. However, the opposite is true as well–there are a lot of qualities that come from ADHD that make for a great spouse. Discover those qualities in your partner and try to work on nurturing them together.

- **Zest for life**. People with ADHD notice so much more than we give them credit for. They notice the little things that we take for granted. They're highly attuned to the world around them. They love to stop and smell the flowers, so to speak. That translates into a huge zest for life and the world around them. They are always finding new ways to appreciate their surroundings or to spruce up their surroundings to bring more joy into your lives. Let them show you how marvelous life can be. Listen when they talk about the wonders they see around them. Hear the passion in their voices as they talk about the things they love. This will give you a new appreciation for life as well.
- **Bravery**. When it comes to bullying, people with the disorder understand what it's like more than almost anyone. They understand what it's like to feel different, to be treated poorly for being different, and to feel as though others don't understand and aren't willing to understand you. They are often the ones rooting for the underdog, the ones who champion justice for others. They're willing to stand up and fight for what they believe in. This means that no one will

ever treat you badly on their watch. Instead, they will look out for you and encourage you to go after what you want, get the justice you deserve when you're wronged, or fight even when the odds seem insurmountable.

- **Spontaneity**. Those with the disorder make for some of the most spontaneously romantic partners because of the desire to experience new things and the craving to shake up the ordinary. You have a good long-term memory which means that you can surprise your spouse with something they mentioned ages ago. It might be tempting to say "no" when they propose a random, wild and crazy adventure but try to go along with it once in a while because you never know what you might get to experience.

- **Creativity**. People with the disorder see the world from a totally unique perspective. They give something their all when they dive into it and can think of many creative, outside-the-box solutions to problems that surprise us. They are fantastically creative and if you can harness that for a moment, you will come up with ideas that are worth listening to. You can encourage your spouse to pick up a creative hobby or outlet for their ideas and watch them blossom. They can plan amazing parties or trips if given a chance and a little support–giving you experiences you never thought possible!

- **Intelligence**. ADHD doesn't necessarily gift people with higher intelligence, but they can see the world uniquely and think of new ways to solve issues, which gives them an edge when it comes to learning new things. When they hyperfocus, they can pick up new skills in a snap. Think about how smart your spouse is and remind them of that when they have some day-to-day difficulties with organization or forgetfulness. They aren't stupid, they just store memory differently, and their brains want to focus on the most interesting thing at the moment. Pull out the puzzles, board games, or trivia games and watch them work. They will amaze you with their pattern recognition and problem-solving.

- **Parenting skills**. People with the disorder are willing to get down on their children's level, join in on their pretend play, and listen to what their kids have to say. They make great hands-on parents who will provide hours of fun and joy for children. Encourage them when it comes to playtime because they can take something mundane and make it fascinating and interesting to your children. They are naturally good at making kids feel heard as well–they understand what it's like to feel passionate about something important.

- **Sense of humor**. Because of the many ways the disorder can affect their daily lives, they have often learned how to cope using humor. They are often extremely funny and clever and make great jokes when you least expect it. They can help keep you grounded by laughing at how silly life can sometimes be, and they can keep you entertained when your spirits are a bit low. Don't be afraid to laugh with them when they laugh at themselves–it helps you both cope with the way the disorder pops up and reminds you that life is too short to take everything so seriously.

- **Kindness**. People with the disorder have an abundance of compassion and empathy for others. They understand what it's like to struggle, go through difficulties, and feel different in a way that makes them stand out to those who would tear them down for it. They love deeply and are very loyal spouses. Embrace their compassion and find a project that the two of you can get into that helps others–give back to your community or ways that you can help others. The two of you will make an unstoppable team when you work together and use your strengths to balance each other out.

There is nothing better than being married to an ADHD-affected spouse—when you learn to look at the good qualities instead of focusing on how the symptoms affect your life. There are so many ways to learn and grow as a couple when you focus on how having an affected marriage can be a good thing.

For one, it helps you accept and understand that life isn't fair and nobody is perfect. Your spouse may drive you crazy, but they are human, just like you. You can embrace your own imperfections as well. Being with an affected spouse gives you the freedom to give up the notion that you can strive for a kind of perfection within–it doesn't exist and you don't need to stress yourself out trying to achieve it. You and your spouse are unique and you have much to offer the world. Your spouse understands more than anyone what it's like to experience unfairness and they can help you out when things get tough and feel like they aren't going your way. Lean on each other and work through those times together.

You will really learn how to work as a team in an affected marriage. You'll notice that there are some things that your partner manages to execute without issue, and some areas in which they struggle. Divide tasks up by your strengths and weaknesses, and you'll realize that so much more is getting done. It doesn't have to be unequal either. There are ways to make it work that still play to your partner's strength, even if they need more encouragement, help, or reminders to get it done. You can combine chores as well. Maybe doing the dishes isn't their forte, but they can help you dry as you wash. The two of you need to learn to work together to accomplish the things that give you both trouble. Divvying up household responsibilities is another way to work together to divide and conquer. If you're better at remembering the household tasks that need doing and your partner is better at managing the household finances, you be in charge of the master schedule and let your partner take over paying bills and planning out your savings.

Sometimes you'll make a mistake. Your spouse is much more likely to understand that most and is more likely to be willing to forgive–they know how it feels to mess up. The more patient you are with them, the more likely they are also to forgive you when you also mess up or break their trust. You will learn forgiveness and compassion for others when in an affected marriage. You will learn that it's pointless to hold onto grudges and that it's unhelpful to stay angry for small missteps. You also learn patience in an affected marriage. Sometimes it takes a dose of patience to deal with someone with the disorder, and you've learned how to become a more patient person overall. That's never a bad thing. You'll have more patience for your own children and your family, you'll become more understanding of people at work that test you or make mistakes–and it's great that you can understand what it's like to feel for others.

The two of you will become awesome communicators. It's vital to be good at communicating when it comes to the disorder because it can often be in-one-ear-out-the-other, through no fault of your spouse. You will learn how to pick your battles, stop reacting when your spouse's anger or frustration gets the better of them, and pick up on the things they *really* mean when they're struggling to communicate with you. The two of you will learn to stop saying things you don't mean because you know that they are a trigger point for arguments and fights–especially because your partner can misinterpret your words. Good communication can be a game-changer when it comes to the disorder; so you will become great at it, in order to work through the issues that crop up. As a result, you two can navigate any situation, even ones that seem hard or impossible, because of how good you are at working together to overcome.

The two of you can become an unstoppable duo of persevering through the tough times. People with the disorder often refuse to let anything stop them when they get passionate about something, and working together, you become an unshakeable force for good. Your spouse wants to succeed at something when they put their mind to it, and when it comes to your marriage, they will do whatever it takes to succeed. You can weather any storm when you have an ADHD spouse because they won't let something small like a tornado tearing your house apart, or getting fired from your job, stop them from making sure that both of you have a good life. Trust and rely on them when times get hard because with their help you can get through anything.

Fostering love and devotion for each other doesn't have to be hard when you can look at the bright side of your relationship. You are with someone who is unique and brings a unique perspective to the world— one that can bless you both in good times and bad. Learning to embrace the good sides of your spouse while letting go of some of the more frustrating aspects will only help the two of you in the long run. And as an affected partner, you can learn to embrace the crazy, absurd, trying times and help your spouse appreciate the good times all the more.

Chapter Summary

- Learning to empathize with each other will help your marriage succeed. You want to see life from your partner's perspective to understand how it's affecting the other person. Listen to what they have to say, try to understand their point of view, and give them grace and compassion as they give you.
- When things seem hard, stressful, or the disorder appears to be making you struggle with your feelings, try to take time for each other so you can fall in love all over again. Make time to spend together, do something new, be spontaneous, and take time for yourselves in order to let yourself miss them and remember the good.
- There are so many positive aspects to having ADHD that make your marriage wonderful. Your spouse is full of compassion, creativity, kindness, and empathy. They can teach you how to be more patient, persevere through the bad, focus on the good, and let go of the trivial.

Conclusion

ADHD affects marriage in numerous ways. It can be difficult to deal with a spouse that has the disorder. Symptoms like trouble paying attention, impulsivity, forgetfulness, emotional dysregulation, difficulty in maintaining relationships, poor organizational skills, difficulty understanding and empathizing with others, and more can affect how the two of you interact and function. You feel as though you're at your wit's end sometimes, and you often feel as though you've taken on a role as more of a parent to your partner than an equal. This can take a toll on your feelings for your partner and can leave you feeling as though you're ready to cut your losses. It's not only on the affected partner, though. The non-affected partner may be contributing by nagging, getting angry or frustrated, infantilizing their partner, berating them, or making them feel guilty or unappreciated.

It doesn't have to be like that, though. The two of you need to understand more about the disorder in order to tackle how to improve it. Studying up on the disorder will help, as will the both of you acknowledging that there is a problem and that problem is affecting the relationship. It's important to recognize the way your disorder is making your partner feel, and it's important that as the non-affected partner, you're acknowledging how your criticism and nagging are making them feel. Start by separating who your partner is from their symptoms. Recognize that they aren't their disorder, that it's a part of them but not the sum of their whole.

Some of the most common relationship problems with ADHD can be solved by learning to work with the disorder instead of against it. Sometimes we want our spouse to just "be normal," but there is no normal with the disorder. You need to put strategies in place to help each other through the problems. Learning how to navigate the disorder will involve becoming more educated about it and figuring out, through trial and error, how to manage the symptoms. You need to put a plan in place to help with navigating chores and household duties and figure out the best strategies to help navigate social situations and understand each other better. Having empathy for the things that your partner goes through as the two of you navigate the symptoms will help you both understand each other better and be more loving and forgiving when things aren't going the way you want or when the disorder is making it difficult to communicate.

Learning how to understand nonverbal cues is one of the best ways that people with the disorder can understand their partner better, especially when we express ourselves a lot through nonverbal means. The two of you can work together to navigate social situations, leading to less frustration, less miscommunication, and less misunderstandings. Having a plan going in will minimize the amount of social blunders that crop up and help your spouse recognize when they're doing things like dominating the conversation or they need some time to recharge. People with the disorder often take criticism and bad experiences to heart, so it's important to be kind when you point out what you want to help your significant other overcome. Conflict will arise, and it's important you know how to navigate it properly. When it comes to discussing sources of conflict, try to be understanding and sympathetic and clear and concise. Your partner will feel shame and embarrassment and may lash out to hide their feelings, but understanding will go a long way towards helping the both of you navigate communication issues.

When your partner feels good about themselves and good about their relationship with you, they're more likely to be open to hearing feedback. Working on your sense of self-identity, separating it from your ADHD, can help you improve self-esteem, which will give you the opportunity to feel secure enough to grow in the relationship. As the non-affected spouse, learning to stand up for yourself and how to say "no" is just as important as gaining self-esteem is to the affected partner. You want to strive for a point where you can put yourself first while still being a considerate partner to your spouse. The goal is to give them a hand while also letting them be independent and feel as though they are your equal.

Though it will be difficult, it will be worth it when you start to see the relationship changes that you've been looking for. You may not know it, but the two of you are starting a very important journey together. You are learning how to accept each other, flaws and all, and how to work together to become a better couple and better friends. Being friends first should be the goal. Treat each other as you would treat your friends and treat each other as you want to be treated. Compliment them when they've done something you appreciate, and make them feel respected, heard, and appreciated. Remember that having the disorder isn't all bad, either. Having ADHD gives people a greater sense of compassion, stronger loyalty, more creativity, and better problem-solving skills. These, when put into effect, can make your spouse into a super-powered spouse, friend, and parent.

It will take more than seven days of work to get there, but using the tips, tricks, and techniques in this book will start your new journey together on the right foot. You have the opportunity to take a good relationship and make it a great one. Don't be scared to talk to each other, lay out what you need going forward, and work together to make that happen. Stumbling blocks will come up, and mistakes will be made along the way, but the two of you are empowered now to make the future exactly how you want it to be.

If you liked this book and found it helpful, please leave a review on Amazon.

Reference

- Rodden, J. & Saline, S. (2022, February 28). What is Executive Dysfunction? Signs and Symptoms of EFD. ADDitude. Retrieved May 12, 2022. From: <u>What Is Executive Dysfunction? Sign and Symptoms of EFD</u>.
- Smith, M. (2021, October). Adult ADHD and Relationships. HelpGuide. Retrieved May 13, 2022. From: <u>Adult ADHD and Relationships - HelpGuide.org</u>
- Halverstadt, J. (2021, January 21). 10 Ways to Save Your Relationships. ADDitude. Retrieved May 12, 2022. From: <u>10 Ways to Save Your Relationship</u>
- Steed, L. (2022, May 5). "You're Not Listening" How ADHD Impulsivity and Insecurity Ruined My Relationship. ADDitude. Retrieved May 6, 2022. From: <u>"You're Not Listening!" How ADHD Impulsivity and Insecurity Ruined My Relationship</u>
- Boyle Wheeler, R. & Bhandari, S. (2020. March 31). Communication Hacks for ADHD. WebMD. Retrieved May 16, 2022. From: <u>Communication Hacks for ADHD</u>
- Smith, J. (2021, June 29). The Secrets to Effectively Manage ADHD and Conflict Resolution. FastBrain. Retrieved May 14, 2022. From: <u>The Secrets to Effectively Manage ADHD and Conflict Resolution– FastBraiin</u>
- Nadeau, K. (n.d.). Building ADHD-friend Relationship Skills as a Couple. Chesapeake Center. Retrieved May 12, 2022. From: <u>Building ADHD-friendly Relationship Skills as a Couple – The Chesapeake Center</u>
- Muggli, L. (2021, January 25). ADHD & Anxiety– Managing the Impact on Relationships. Laura Muggli. Retrieved May 14, 2022. From: <u>ADHD & Anxiety - Managing the Impact on Relationships</u>
- Broadbent, E. (2021, June 24). We Need to Talk About How ADHD Affects Interpersonal Relationships. ADDitude. Retrieved May 12, 2022. From: <u>We Need to Talk About How ADHD Affects Interpersonal Relationships</u>

- Amen, D. (2020, July 28). Why We Crave the Drama That Sabotages Relationships. ADDitude. Retrieved May 14, 2022. From: <u>Why We Crave the Drama That Sabotages Relationships</u>
- Jaska, P. (2021, July 22). How to Regain Your Confidence: Life-Changing Strategies for Adults with ADHD. ADDitude. Retrieved May 18, 2022. From: <u>How to Regain Your Confidence: Life-Changing Strategies for Adults with ADHD</u>

CPSIA information can be obtained
at www.ICGtesting.com
Printed in the USA
LVHW080724090922
727942LV00008B/391